Practical Manual of HISTOLOGY *for Medical Students*

Practical Manual of HISTOLOGY *for Medical Students*

Second Edition

Neelkanth Kote

Author & Healthcare Service Organizer
Secretary of RRMCH Alumni Association
Rajarajeswari Medical College and Hospital (RRMCH)
Bengaluru, Karnataka, India
Email: kote.neelkanthb@gmail.com

Foreword

DL Ramachandra

JAYPEE The Health Sciences Publishers

New Delhi | London | Philadelphia | Panama

Jaypee Brothers Medical Publishers (P) Ltd

Headquarters

Jaypee Brothers Medical Publishers (P) Ltd
4838/24, Ansari Road, Daryaganj
New Delhi 110 002, India
Phone: +91-11-43574357
Fax: +91-11-43574314
Email: jaypee@jaypeebrothers.com

Overseas Offices

J.P. Medical Ltd
83 Victoria Street, London
SW1H 0HW (UK)
Phone: +44 20 3170 8910
Fax: +44 (0)20 3008 6180
Email: info@jpmedpub.com

Jaypee-Highlights Medical Publishers Inc
City of Knowledge, Bld. 237, Clayton
Panama City, Panama
Phone: +1 507-301-0496
Fax: +1 507-301-0499
Email: cservice@jphmedical.com

Jaypee Medical Inc
The Bourse
111 South Independence Mall East
Suite 835, Philadelphia, PA 19106, USA
Phone: +1 267-519-9789
Email: jpmed.us@gmail.com

Jaypee Brothers Medical Publishers (P) Ltd
17/1-B Babar Road, Block-B, Shaymali
Mohammadpur, Dhaka-1207
Bangladesh
Mobile: +08801912003485
Email: jaypeedhaka@gmail.com

Jaypee Brothers Medical Publishers (P) Ltd
Bhotahity, Kathmandu, Nepal
Phone +977-9741283608
Email: kathmandu@jaypeebrothers.com

Website: www.jaypeebrothers.com
Website: www.jaypeedigital.com

Inquiries for bulk sales may be solicited at: jaypee@jaypeebrothers.com

Practical Manual of Histology for Medical Students

First Edition: 2009

Second Edition: ***2014***

ISBN 978-93-5152-391-8

Printed at: Samrat Offset Pvt. Ltd.

Dedicated to

My parents
Smt Jaisheela B Kote
Sri Basavaraj V Kote
and
The entire Kote family
for their eternal love, care and
affection towards me.

Foreword

Rajarajeswari Medical College and Hospital
Kambipura, Near Kengeri Hobli, Mysore Road, Bengaluru - 560 074
Ph.: 080-65661805 Fax: 080-28437393

(Approved by Medical Council of India and Government of India and
Affiliated to Rajiv Gandhi University of Health Sciences, Bengaluru)
Sponsored by:

MOOGAMBIGAI CHARITABLE AND EDUCATIONAL TRUST

The author deserves to be congratulated for presenting to the medical students an easy access to the subject of Anatomy (Histology). With lots of passion and great efforts, he has been able to put through in the book the quantum of knowledge that is to be imparted in the ever-growing specialty—Histology.

He has defined the structure of different organs of the human body with attractive pictures. The language is simple and easily understandable. The students will greatly benefit by the descriptive account of Histology in Anatomy.

I am sure this book will be welcomed by the students of Anatomy at all levels including Dental, Nursing and others.

I am confident that this book will go through many editions in the coming years with more details.

DL Ramachandra MD FIMS
Medical Director
Rajarajeswari Medical College and Hospital (RRMCH)
Bengaluru, Karnataka, India

Preface to the Second Edition

First of all I would like to thank all my dear students for accepting the book with an open mind. It gives me an immense sense of satisfaction when I get the feedback from students of different medical colleges. Thank you all for your honest comments and suggestions.

With a new hope of making histology more easier for medical students I have made slight changes and the good old concepts of first edition are retained same for your convenience.

The salient features of second edition of the book are:

- Updated color atlas of histology with identification points
- Photographic pictures of each slide with hand-drawn diagrams of good quality, for correlation
- A special concentration on all the important examination slides with three identification points for each
- Increase in the size of the book for better reading
- Advanced graphics and printing skills for good visualization and understanding of the concepts
- Useful for both theory and practical examinations by universities

I hope the second edition of the book will provide you a better knowledge in understanding the concepts of histology with less burden of study during examination. Please feel free to mail me your valuable comments and suggestions.

Thank you

Neelkanth Kote
Email: kote.neelkanthb@gmail.com

Preface to the First Edition

Dear Students,

I am very happy to share with you that the *Practical Manual of Histology for Medical Students*, a 3-year-old dream of mine has finally come true with the support of Jaypee Brothers Medical Publishers (P) Ltd and its staff.

This book has most of the aspects of the practical Histology, which an undergraduate medical student requires to have. However, this book is not written to replace any other standard books of Histology.

I have tried my level best to make Histology easier for students by considering the difficulties that were faced by me, while I was studying Histology and lots of efforts have been put forward to write this book with a great passion.

A special care has been taken to ensure the quality and clarity of the matter, and a great support from my friends and juniors have made me to focus on my book project continuously till the end.

The salient features of this book are:

- Brief specific explanation in points with an easy and palatable language
- Easily understandable and attractive handy diagrams by the students
- Three identification points for all the examination slides
- A special concentration on all the important examination slides
- Introduction of Clinical Histology part, which makes the subject more interesting
- Discussion containing the list of important probable questions asked by the examiners during slide discussion
- A color atlas with three identification points, which help the students to go through all the examination slides just before the practical examination.

Hope, the book satisfies the demands of all the medical students in Histology as that is our prime motto of releasing the book.

Still I am a growing bud in this career, so I require your support and cooperation to improve the book quality. Any suggestions and comments are most welcome.

Thank you

Neelkanth Kote
Email: kote.neelkanthb@gmail.com

Acknowledgments

I would like to thank:

Dr Ramachandra, Medical Director of Rajarajeswari Medical College and Hospital (RRMCH), Bengaluru, Karnataka, India, for his encouragement and moral support.

HOD and all the staff of Department of Anatomy, RRMCH, for their valuable suggestions and cooperation.

My special thanks to Dr Balasubramanyam V, Professor of Anatomy, St Johns Medical College, Bengaluru, Karnataka, India, and Dr Balakrishna, Professor of Anatomy, RRMCH, as without their advice and guidance the second edition of the book would have been incomplete.

Shri Jitendar P Vij (Group Chairman), Mr Ankit Vij (Group-President), Mr Tarun Duneja (Director–Publishing) and Mr Venugopal Vishnumurthy [General Manager-Sales & Marketing (South)], Bengaluru of M/s Jaypee Brothers Medical Publishers (P) Ltd, New Delhi, India, for their great support and endeavor in this project.

Mrs Sajini SV (Team Head) and all staff of Bengaluru Production Unit of M/s Jaypee Brothers Medical Publishers (P) Ltd, Bengaluru, for their dedicated work in giving new image and quality standards to the book.

Finally the due love, affection, respect and honor to my parents, sisters, relatives and friends who played an important part to bring charm and glory to my work.

Contents

LIST OF EXAMINATION SLIDES

General Histology

Systemic Histology

SECTION 1

Introduction

CHAPTER 1

Color Atlas with Identification Points

1. **Loose areolar connective tissue (Fig. 6.12A)**
   - Long wavy collagen fibers
   - Short branching elastic fibers
   - Different types of connective tissue cells.

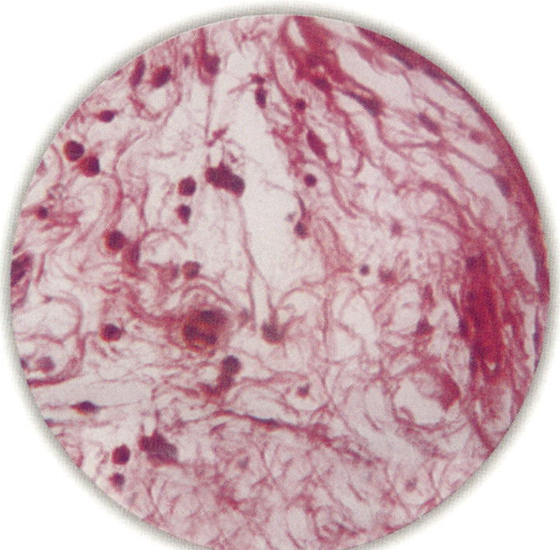

A

2. **Adipose tissue (Fig. 6.13A)**
   - Rounded/Oval/Polygonal cells
   - Lobules with interlobular septum
   - Signet ring appearance.

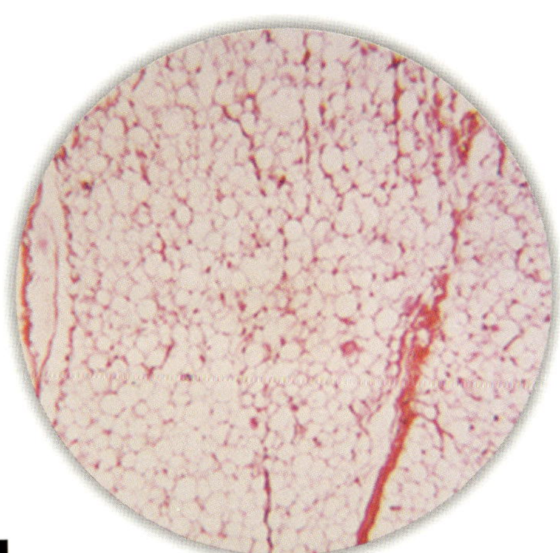

A

3. **Compact bone [Transverse section (TS)] (Fig. 7.2A)**
   - Presence of haversian system
   - Haversian canal containing blood vessels
   - Different types of lamellae.

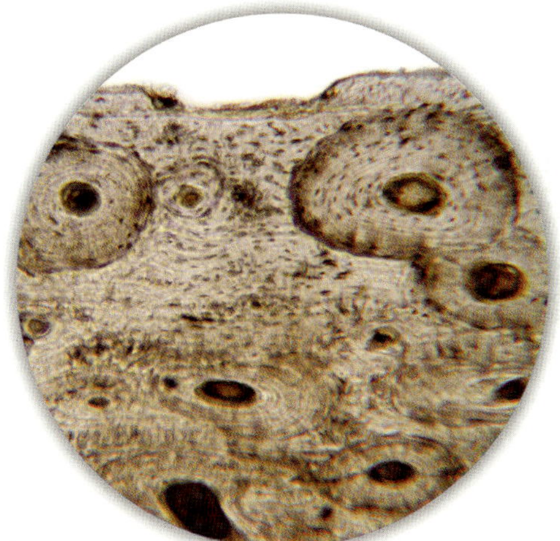

A

4. **Compact bone [Longitudinal section (LS)] (Fig. 7.3A)**
   - Longitudinal sections of haversian canal
   - Horizontal sections of Volk mann's canal
   - Lamellae parallel to haversian canal.

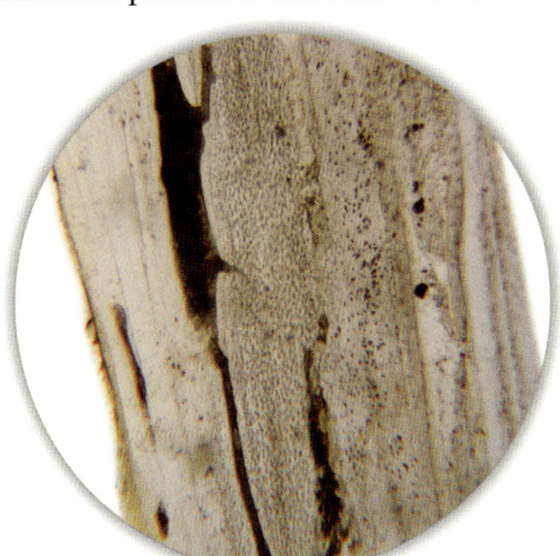

A

5. **Hyaline cartilage (Fig. 7.7A)**
   - Outermost perichondrium
   - Homogeneous matrix
   - Chondrocytes forming cell nests.

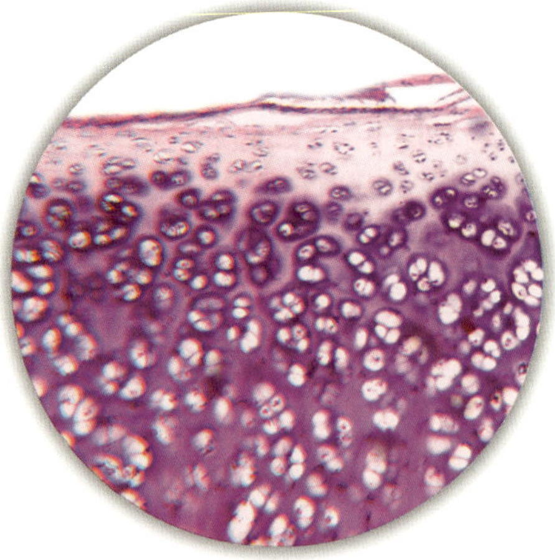

A

6. **Elastic cartilage (Fig. 7.8A)**
   - Outermost perichondrium
   - Matrix rich in elastic fibers
   - Numerous chondrocytes in matrix.

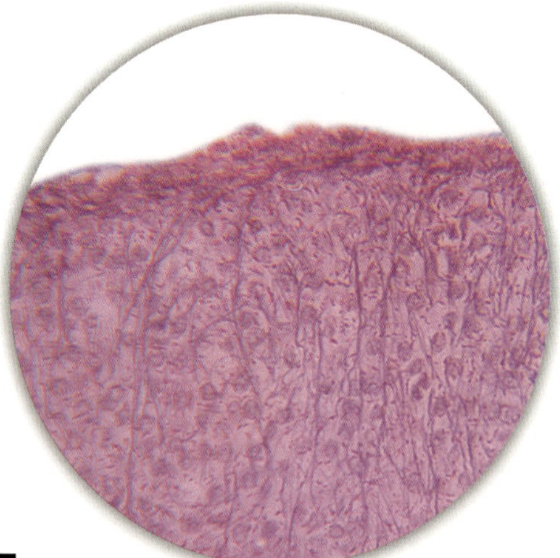

A

7. **White fibrocartilage (Fig. 7.9A)**
   - Absence of perichondrium
   - Matrix rich in collagen fibers
   - Very few chondrocytes arranged in rows.

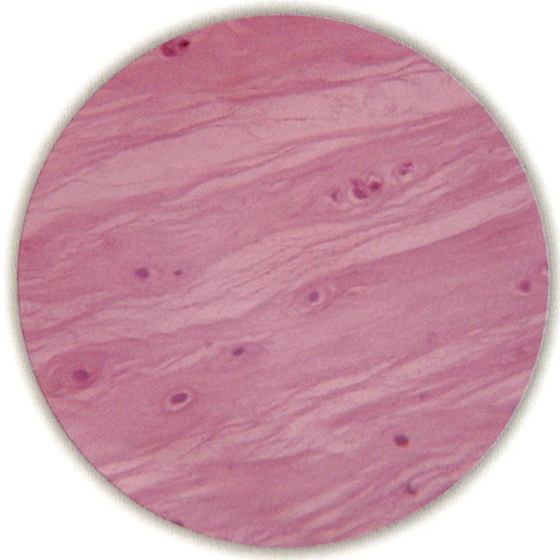

A

8. **Skeletal muscle (LS) (Fig. 8.2A)**
   - Long cylindrical muscle cells
   - Alternative dark and light bands
   - Multinuclei at the periphery.

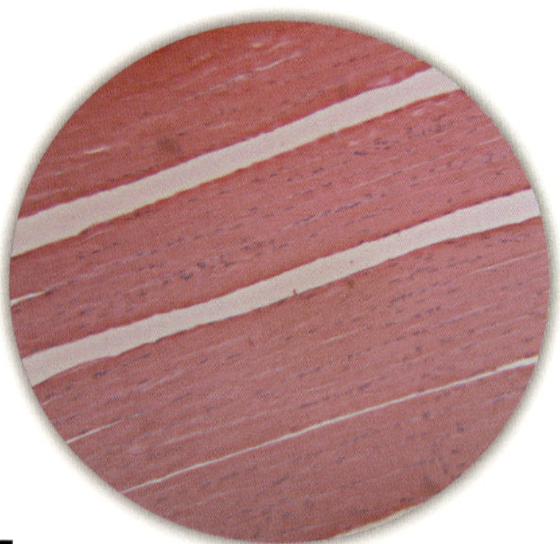

A

9. Skeletal muscle (TS) (Fig. 8.3A)

- Peripherally nucleated muscle bundles or fascicles
- Perimysium around the muscle fascicles
- Epimysium covering the whole muscle tissue.

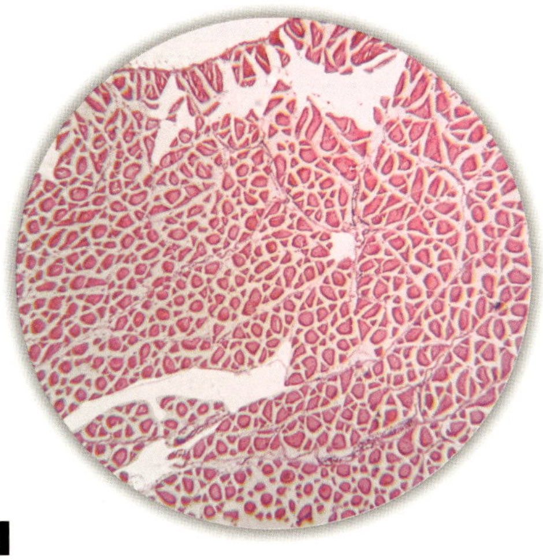

A

11. Cardiac muscle (LS) (Fig. 8.5A)

- Long cylindrical muscle fibers
- Centrally place nucleus
- Presence of intercalated disks.

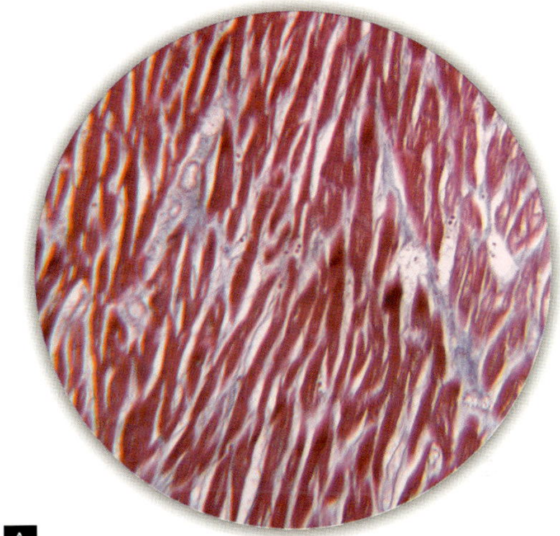

A

10. Smooth muscle (LS) (Fig. 8.4)

- Long spindle-shaped myocytes in bundle
- Absence of striations
- Central flat oval nucleus.

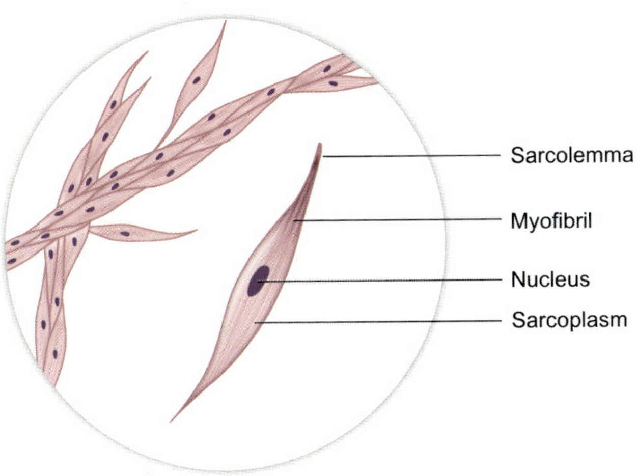

12. Peripheral nerve (LS) (Fig. 9.3A)

- Long cylindrical nerve fibers
- Central axon with myelin sheath
- Presence of nodes of Ranvier.

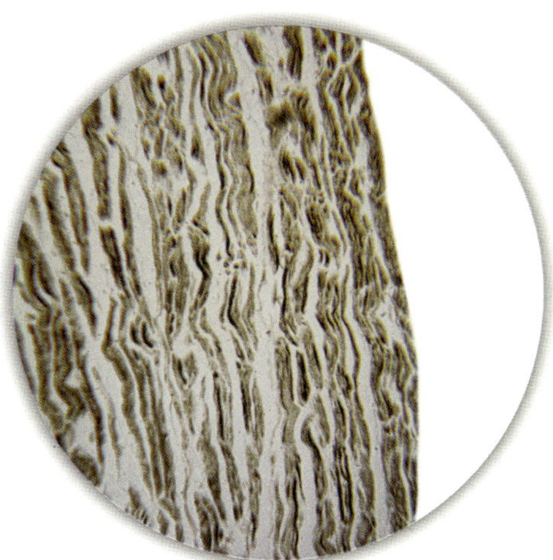

A

13. Peripheral nerve (TS) (Fig. 9.4A)
- Nerve fibers arranged in fascicles
- Perineurium covering the fascicles
- Epineurium covering the whole nerve.

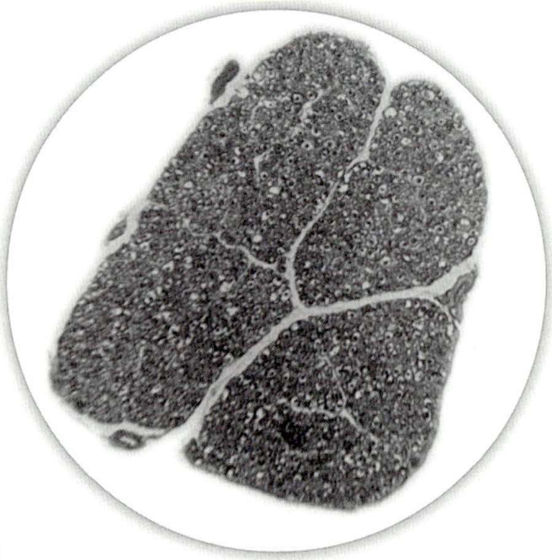

A

14. Spinal ganglion (Fig. 9.5)
- Large pseudounipolar neurons
- Neurons with centrally placed nuclei
- Well-described satellite cells.

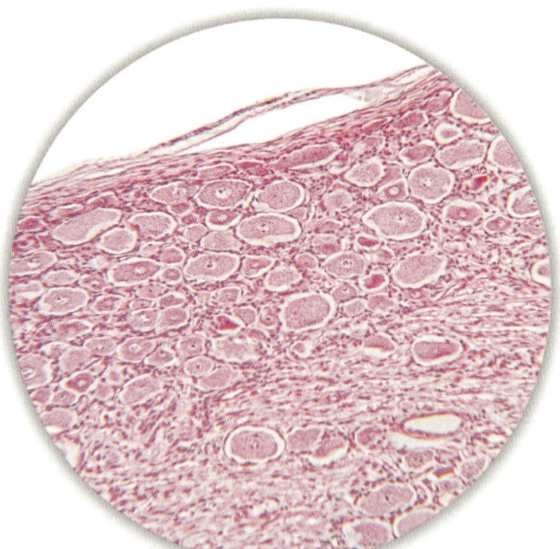

15. Sympathetic ganglion (Fig. 9.6)
- Small multipolar neurons
- Neurons with eccentrically placed nuclei
- Poorly defined satellite cells.

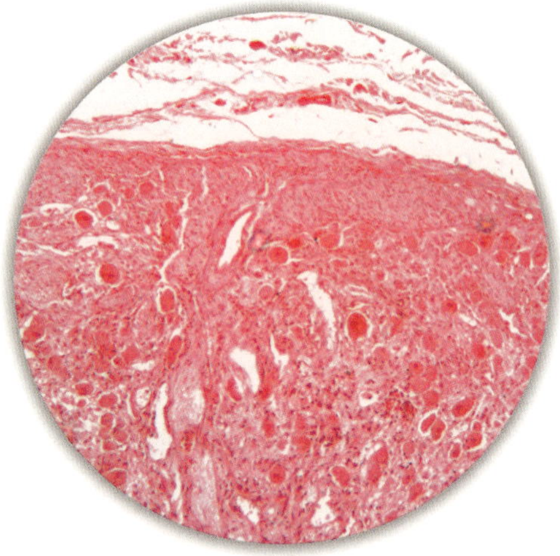

16. Lymph node (Fig. 10.1A)
- Subcapsular sinus or space
- Cortex showing lymphatic nodules
- Medulla rich in blood vessels.

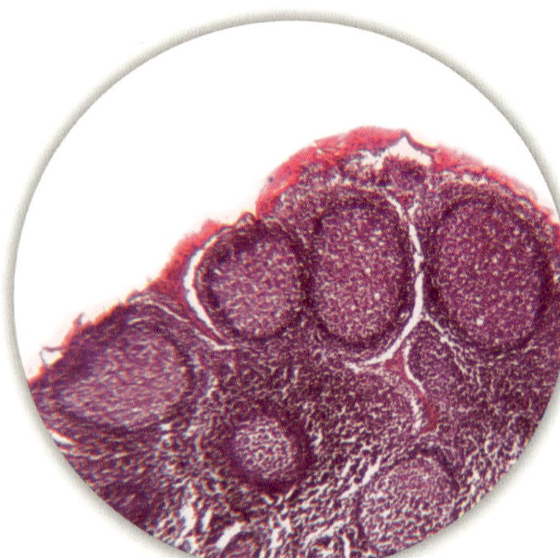

A

17. Spleen (Fig. 10.2A)

- Outermost capsule with trabeculae
- White pulp with eccentrically placed arteriole
- Red pulp rich in blood sinusoids.

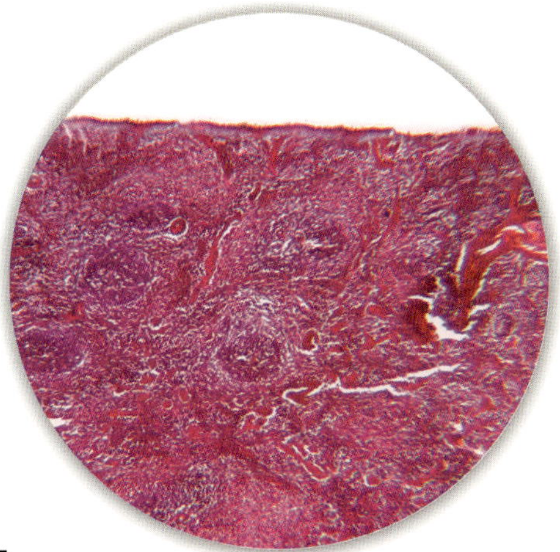

A

18. Thymus (Fig. 10.3A)

- Outermost capsule with incomplete septae
- Lobules with cortex and medulla
- Hassall's corpuscles in medulla.

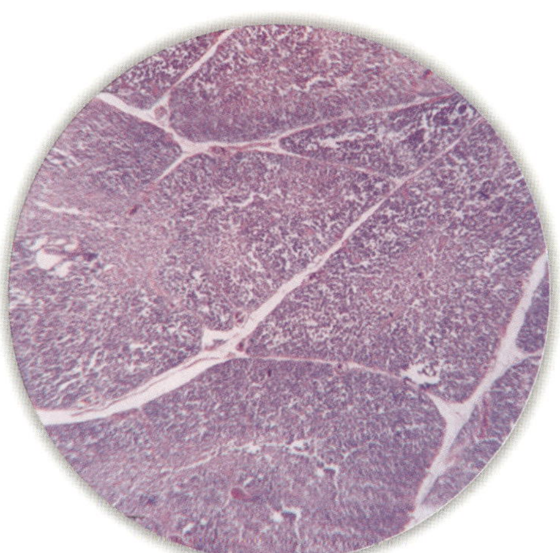

A

19. Palatine tonsil (Fig. 10.4A)

- Deep tonsillar crypts
- Stratified squamous non-keratinized epithelium lining the surface
- Lymphatic nodules with germinal center.

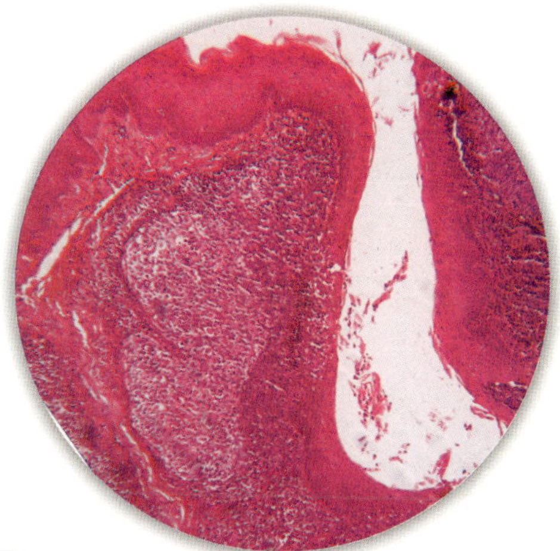

A

20. Large artery (Fig. 11.2A)

- Circular lumen
- Thick tunica media rich in elastic fibers
- Vasa vasorum in tunica adventitia.

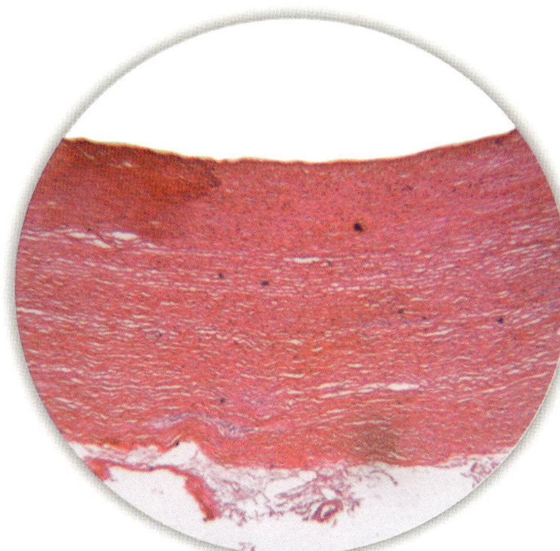

A

21. Medium size artery (Fig. 11.3A)

- Circular lumen
- Prominent internal elastic lamina
- Tunica media rich in circular smooth muscles.

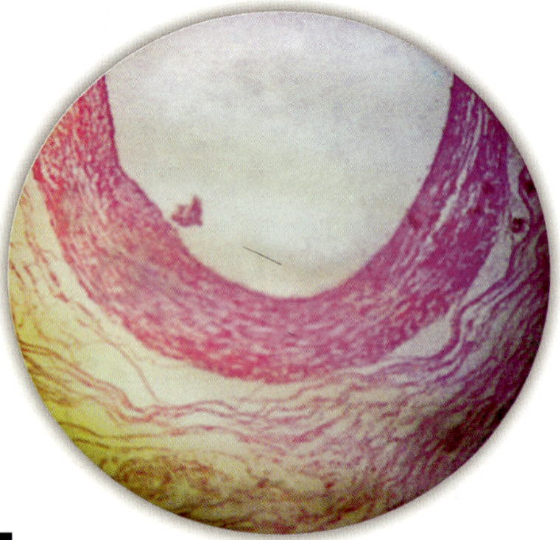

A

22. Large size vein (Fig. 11.6A)

- Collapsed lumen
- Thin tunica media with circular muscle fibers
- Thick tunica adventitia with longitudinal smooth muscles and vasa vasorum.

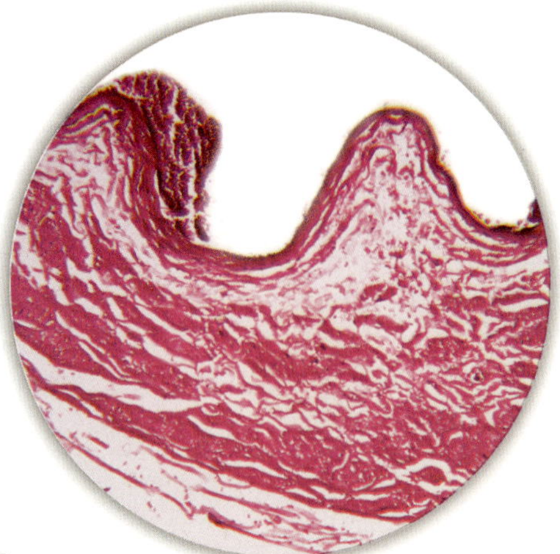

A

23. Medium size vein (Fig. 11.7A)

- Collapsed lumen
- Tunica media containing circular smooth muscles
- Tunica adventitia with dense irregular connective tissue.

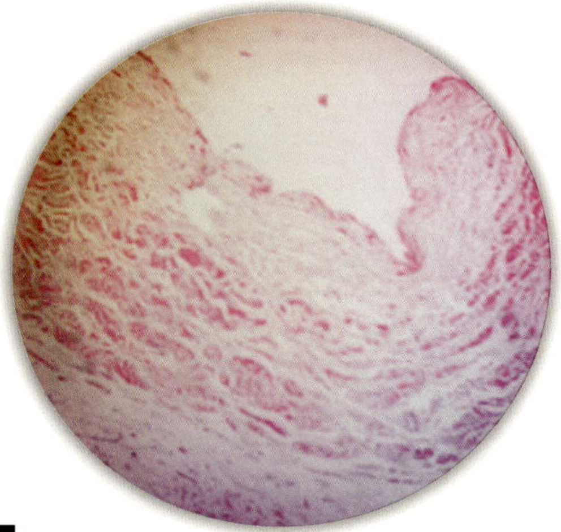

A

24. Thick skin (Fig. 12.3A)

- Thick epidermis of stratified squamous keratinized epithelium
- Prominent dermal and epidermal papillae
- Absence of hair follicles.

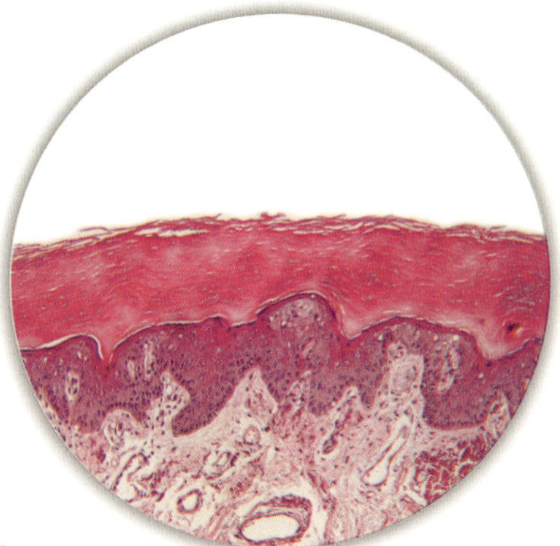

A

25. Thin skin (Fig. 12.4A)

- Thin epidermis of stratified squamous non-keratinized epithelium
- Unmarked dermal and epidermal papillae
- Hair follicles with sebaceous glands and arrector pili muscles.

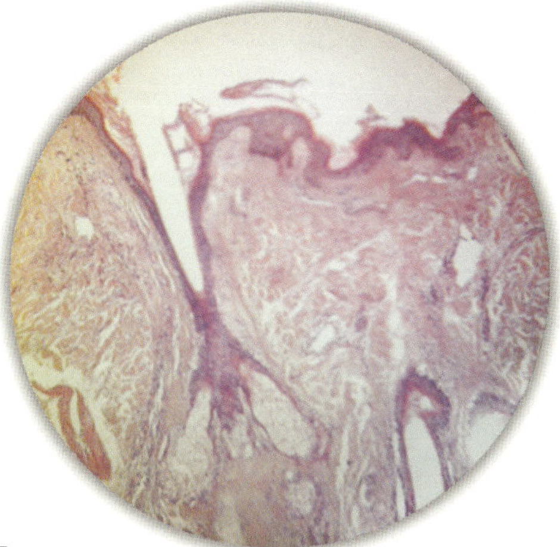

A

26. Circumvallate papilla (Fig. 13.2A)

- Lined by stratified squamous non-keratinized epithelium
- Numerous taste buds in the groove
- Presence of serous glands of von Ebner.

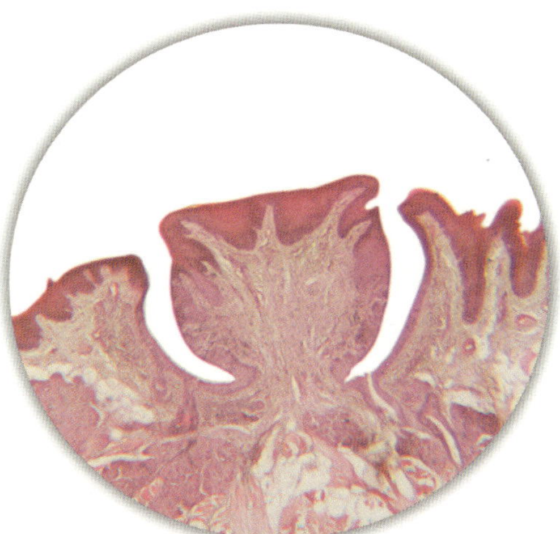

A

27. Filiform papilla (Fig. 13.3A)

- Finger-shaped structure
- Lined by stratified squamous keratinized epithelium
- Skeletal muscle protruding its substance.

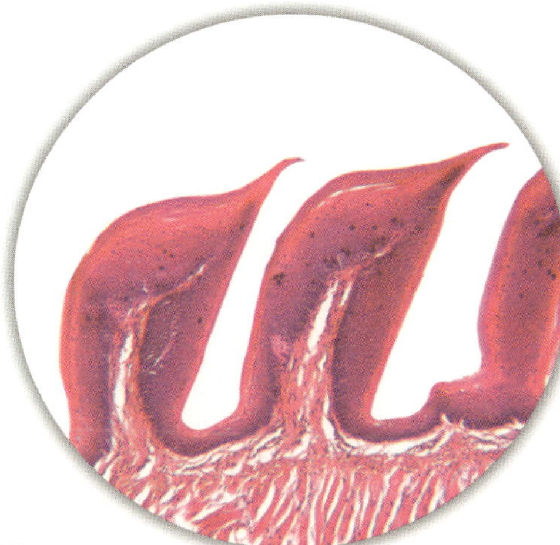

A

28. Fungiform papilla (Fig. 13.4A)

- Mushroom-shaped structure
- Lined by stratified squamous non-keratinized epithelium
- Skeletal muscle protruding its substance.

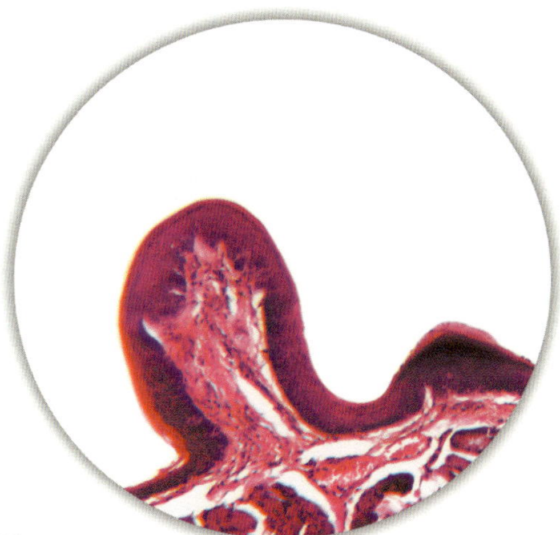

A

29. Parotid salivary gland (Fig. 14.2A)
- Serous acini with narrow lumen
- Centrally placed round nuclei
- Numerous ducts are present.

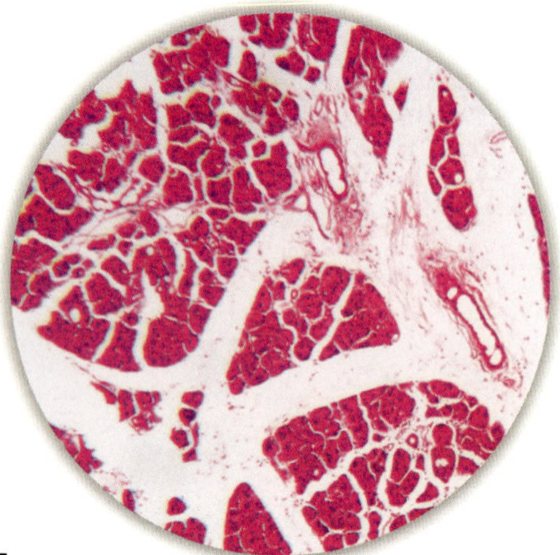

A

30. Sublingual salivary gland (Fig. 14.3A)
- Mucous acini with a large lumen
- Flat nucleus placed near the base of the cell
- Very few ducts are present.

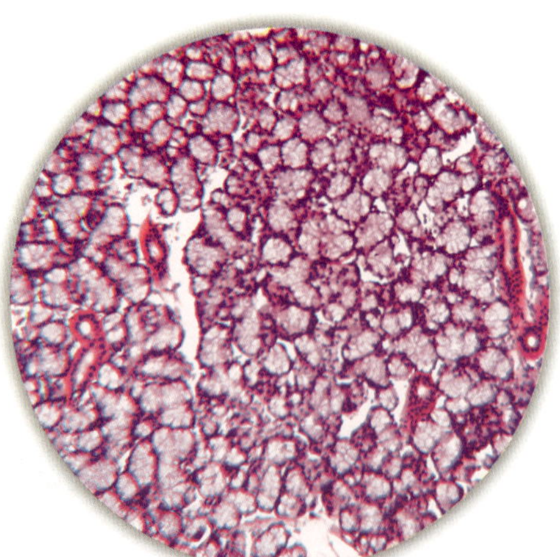

A

31. Submandibular salivary gland (Fig. 14.4A)
- Both serous and mucous acini are seen
- Serous demilunes of Gianuzzi are present
- Few ducts are present.

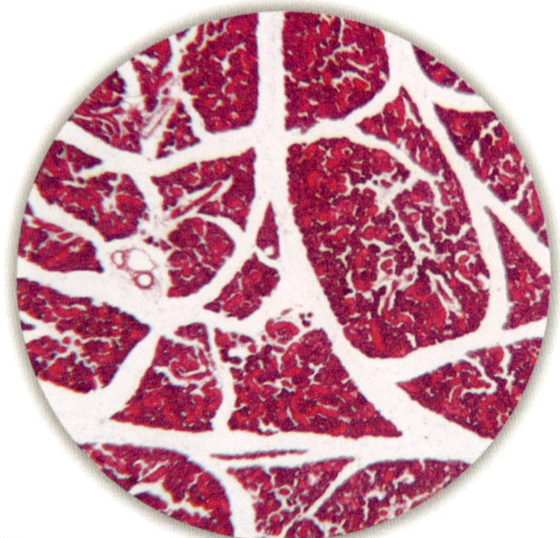

A

32. Esophagus (TS) (Fig. 15.1A)
- Mucosa lined by stratified squamous non-keratinized epithelium
- Submucosa containing esophageal glands
- Muscularis externa containing inner circular and outer longitudinal muscle layer.

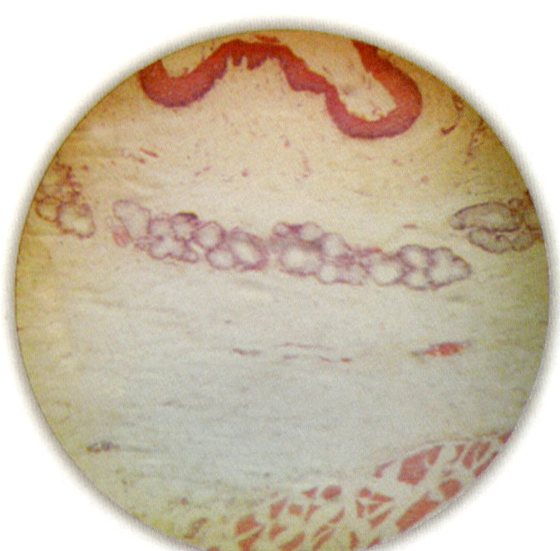

A

33. Stomach (Fundus) (TS) (Fig. 15.2A)

- Mucosa lined by simple columnar epithelium
- Numerous chief and parietal cells in lamina propria
- Muscularis externa containing inner oblique, middle circular and outer longitudinal muscle layer.

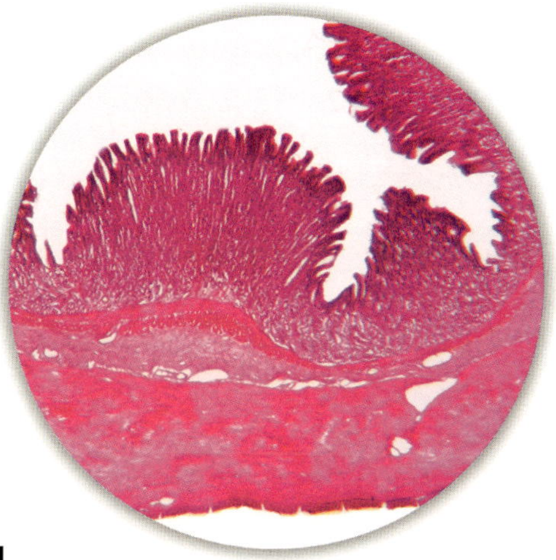

A

35. Duodenum (TS) (Fig. 16.2A)

- Numerous villi
- Crypts of Lieberkühn present
- Brunner's glands in submucosa.

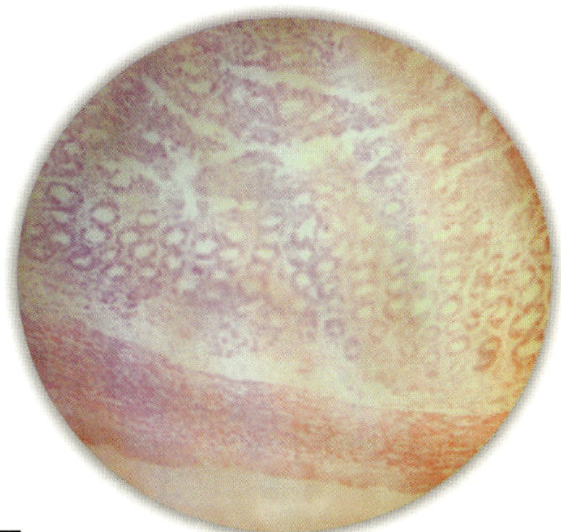

A

34. Stomach (Pylorus) (TS) (Fig. 15.3A)

- Deep gastric pits
- Lamina propria containing pyloric glands
- Thickened middle circular muscle layer forming pyloric sphincter.

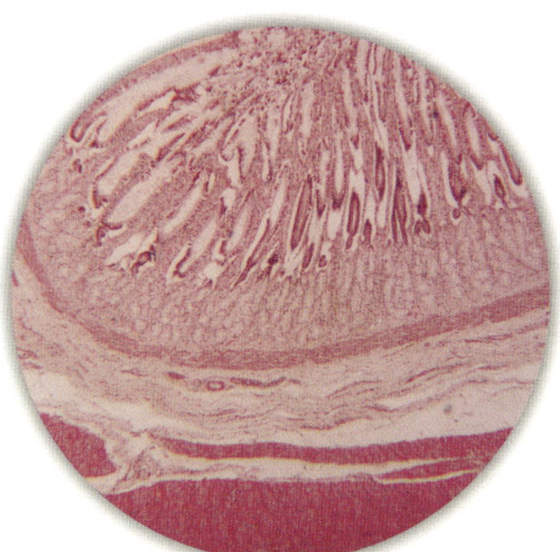

A

36. Jejunum (TS) (Fig. 16.3A)

- Tall villi lined by simple columnar epithelium with goblet cells
- Absence of Brunner's glands in submucosa
- Absence of Peyer's patches.

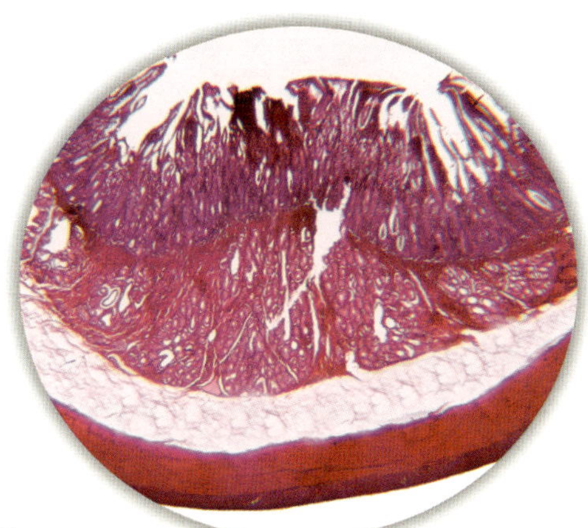

A

37. Ileum (TS) (Fig. 16.4A)

- Small villi rich in goblet cells
- Crypts of Lieberkühn present
- Mucosa containing Peyer's patches.

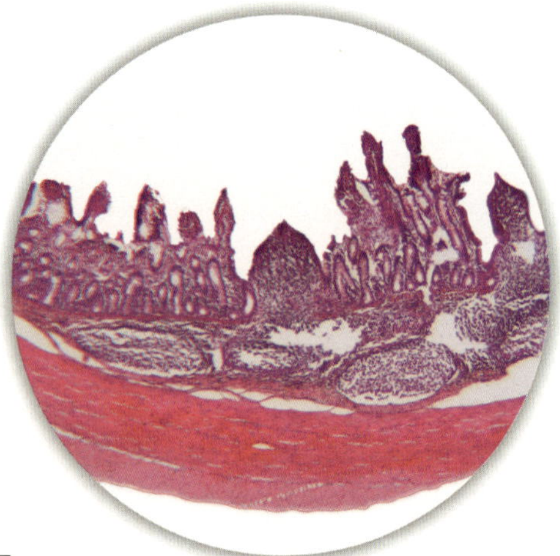

A

39. Colon (TS) (Fig. 16.6A)

- Mucosa with folds, but no villi
- Numerous goblets cells
- Prominent teniae coli.

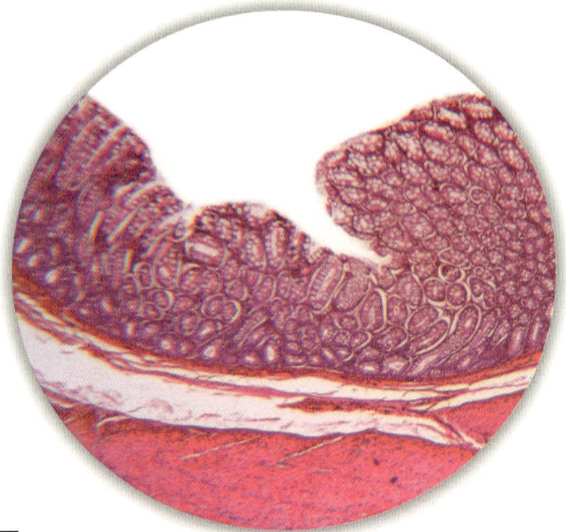

A

38. Vermiform appendix (TS) (Fig. 16.5A)

- Villi are absent
- Lamina propria containing lymphoid aggregations
- Thick muscular layer.

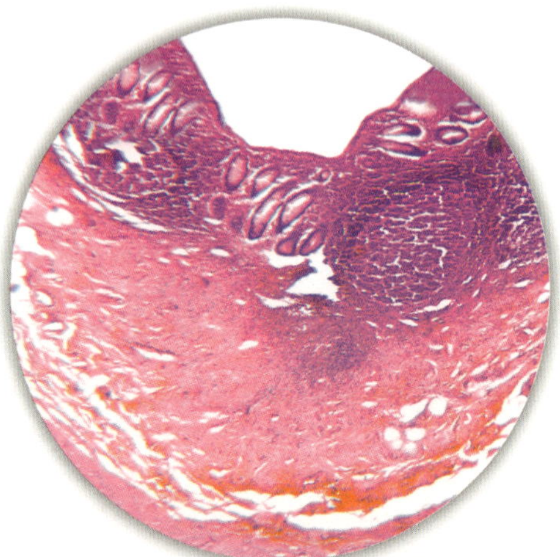

A

40. Pancreas (Fig. 16.7A)

- Numerous serous acini
- Islets of Langerhans are present
- Interlobular ducts are seen.

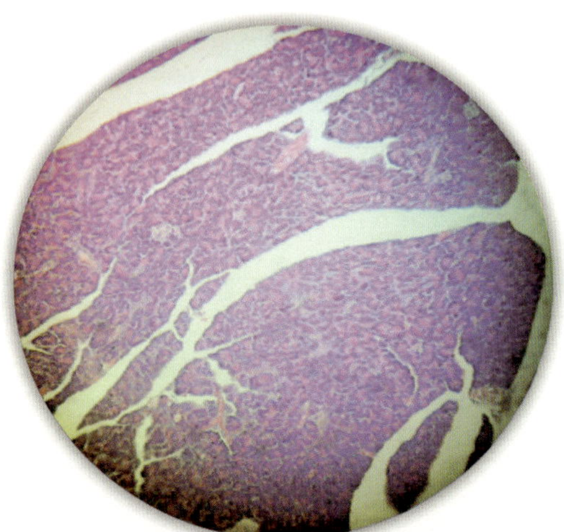

A

41. Liver (Fig. 17.1A)

- Hepatic lobules with central vein
- Radiating hepatic cord cells
- Portal triad is seen.

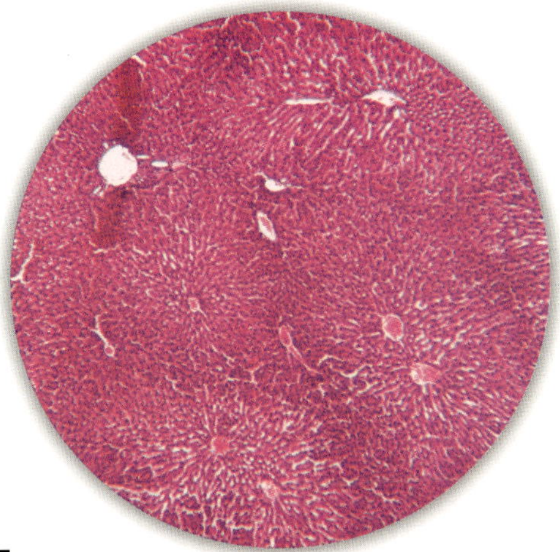

A

42. Gallbladder (Fig. 17.4A)

- Honeycomb appearance of mucosa
- Absence of submucosa and muscularis mucosa
- Presence of fibromuscular coat.

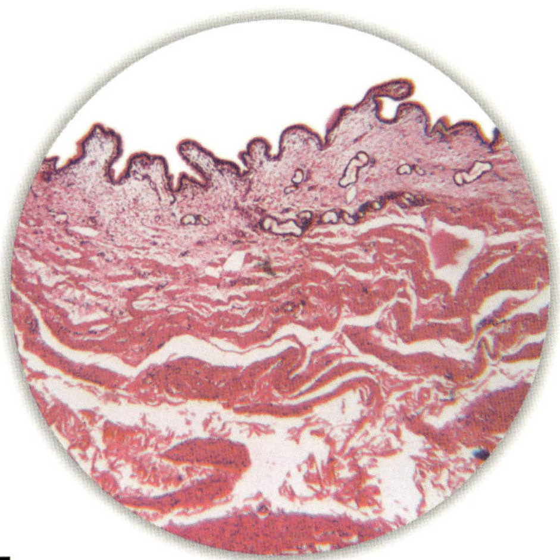

A

43. Kidney (Fig. 18.2A)

- Outer cortex and inner medulla
- Cortex containing renal corpuscles, proximal and distal convoluted tubules
- Medulla containing Henle's loop and collecting ducts.

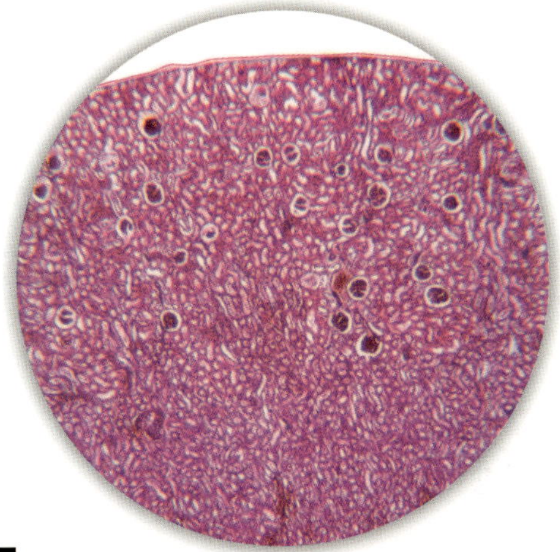

A

44. Ureter (TS) (Fig. 18.4A)

- Star-shaped lumen
- Mucosa lined by transitional epithelium
- Inner longitudinal and outer circular muscle coat present.

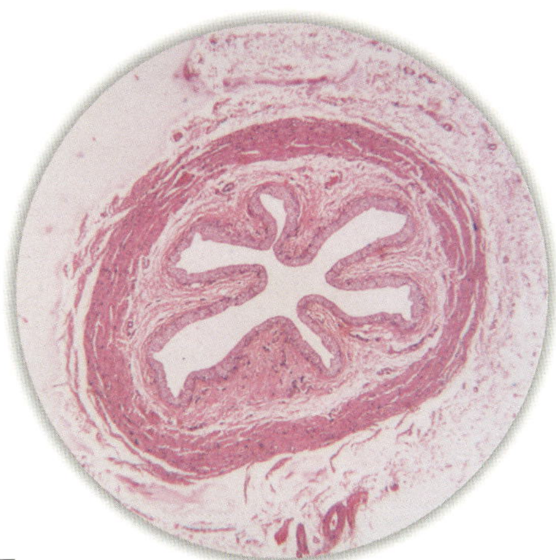

A

45. Urinary bladder (TS) (Fig. 18.5A)

- Mucosa lined by transitional epithelium
- Submucosa is absent
- Muscular layer containing detrusor muscles.

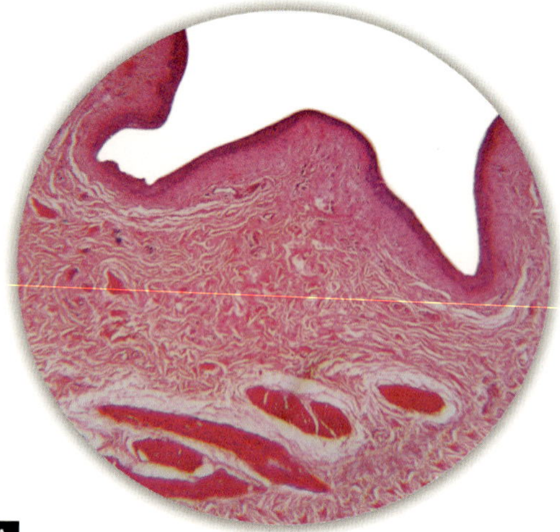

A

47. Lung (Fig. 19.3A)

- Honeycomb appearance of alveoli
- Simple squamous epithelium lining the pulmonary alveoli
- Intrapulmonary bronchi, bronchioles and respiratory bronchioles are seen.

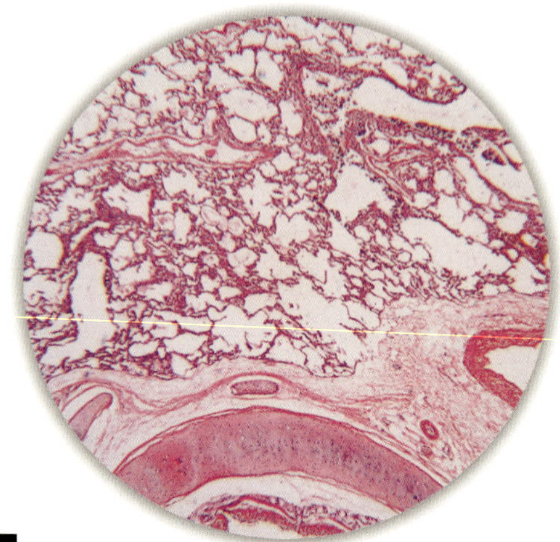

A

46. Trachea (TS) (Fig. 19.2A)

- Mucosa lined by pseudostratified ciliated columnar epithelium with goblet cells
- Submucosa containing serous and mucous glands
- Hyaline cartilaginous ring.

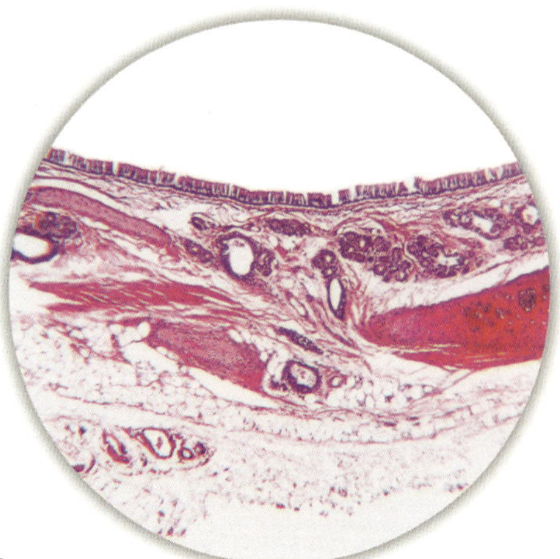

A

48. Pituitary gland (Fig. 20.1A)

- Pars anterior rich in cells and sinusoids
- Interglandular cleft with few colloidal vesicles
- Pars posterior rich in pituicytes and nerve fibers.

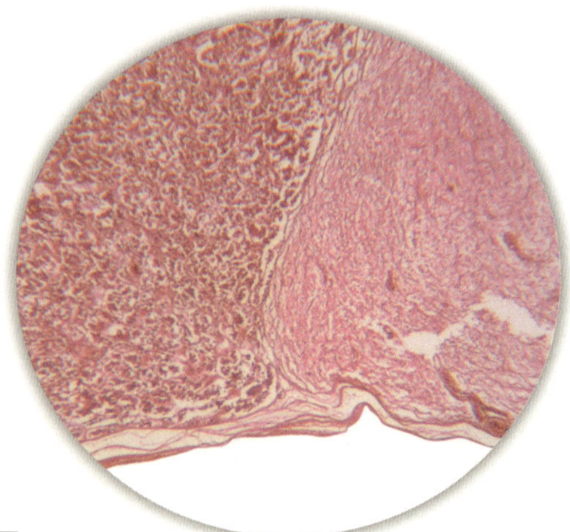

A

49. Thyroid gland (Fig. 20.4A)

- Thyroid follicles lined by cuboidal epithelium
- Eosinophilic colloid in follicular cavity
- Parafollicular cells are seen.

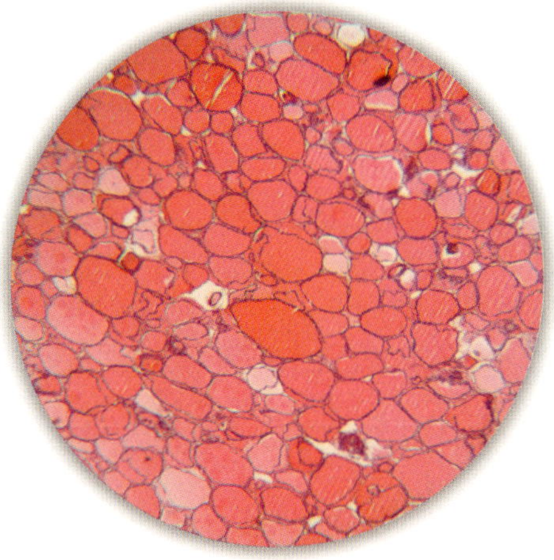

A

50. Parathyroid gland (Fig. 20.5A)

- Irregular cords of chief cells
- Large eosinophilic oxyphil cells
- Thyroid gland may be the accompanying structure.

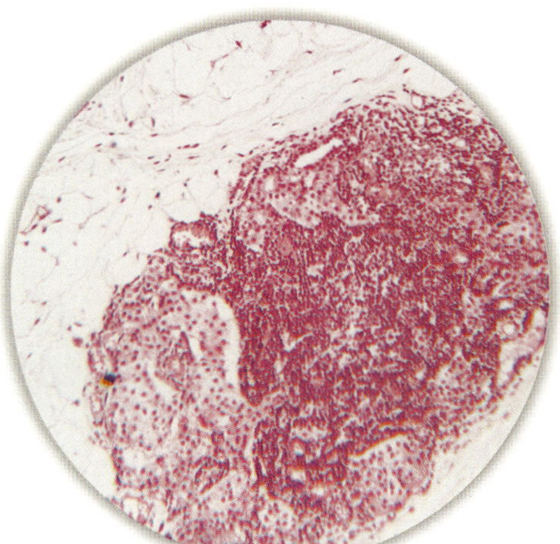

A

51. Suprarenal gland (Fig. 20.7A)

- Outermost capsule with trabeculae
- Cortex showing zona glomerulosa, fasiculata and reticularis
- Medulla showing sinusoids and sympathetic ganglion cells.

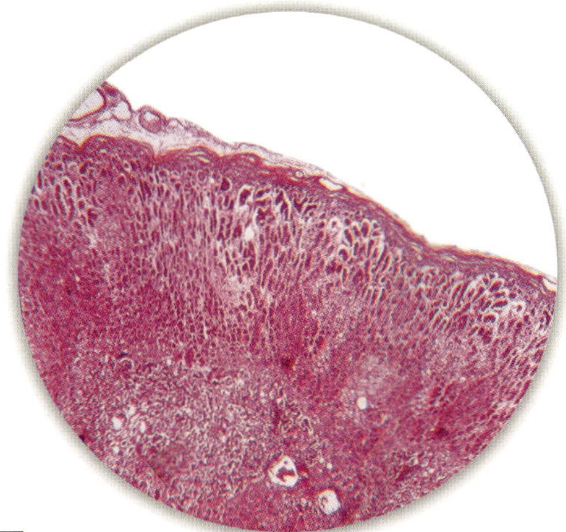

A

52. Testis (Fig. 21.2A)

- Numerous seminiferous tubules
- Interstitial cells of Leydig present
- Sertoli cells in seminiferous epithelium.

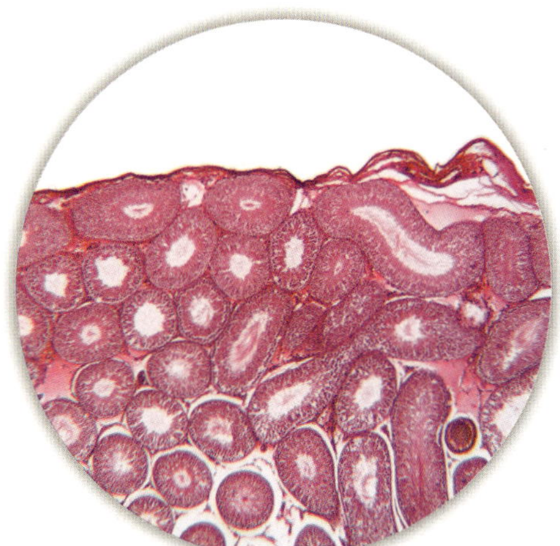

A

53. Epididymis (TS) (Fig. 21.5A)

- Tubules lined by pseudostratified columnar epithelium
- Sperms in the tubular lumen
- Thin circular muscle layer surrounding the ducts.

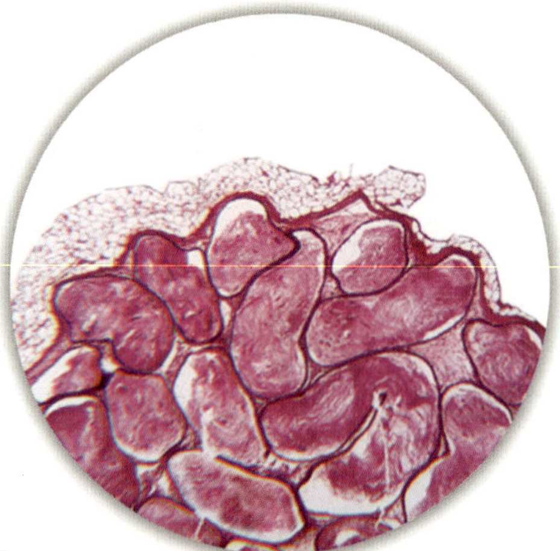

A

55. Seminal vesicle (Fig. 21.8A)

- Branching and anastomosing mucosal folds
- Mucosa lined by pseudostratified columnar epithelium
- Muscular coat of inner circular muscle and outer longitudinal muscles.

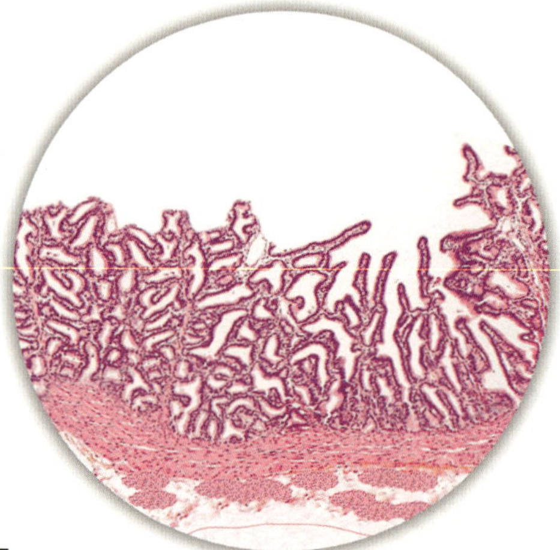

A

54. Vas deferens (TS) (Fig. 21.6A)

- Small stellate lumen
- Lined by pseudostratified ciliated columnar epithelium
- Thick muscle coat of inner longitudinal, middle circular and outer longitudinal layer.

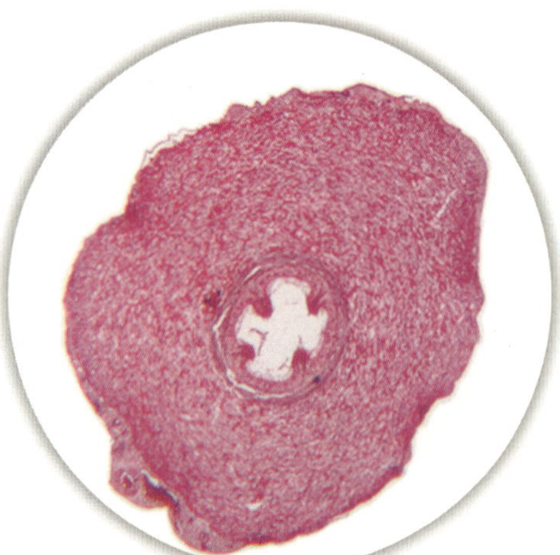

A

56. Prostate (Fig. 21.9A)

- Prostatic acini, lined by simple columnar epithelium
- Fibromuscular stroma
- Corpora amylacea in the lumen.

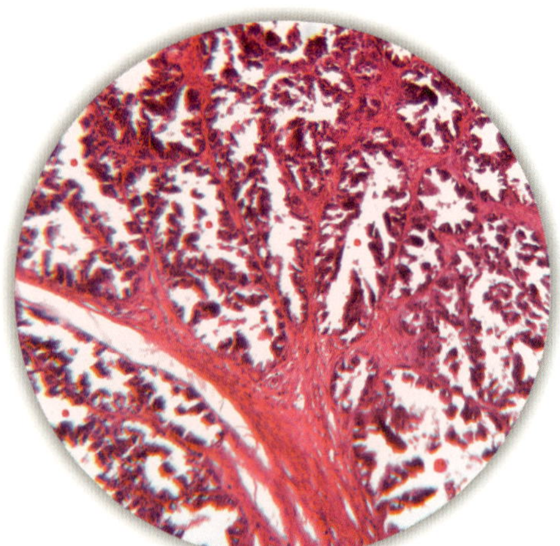

A

57. Ovary (Fig. 22.2A)

- Tunica albuginea with germinal epithelium
- Cortex showing ovarian follicles of different stages
- Medulla showing blood vessels.

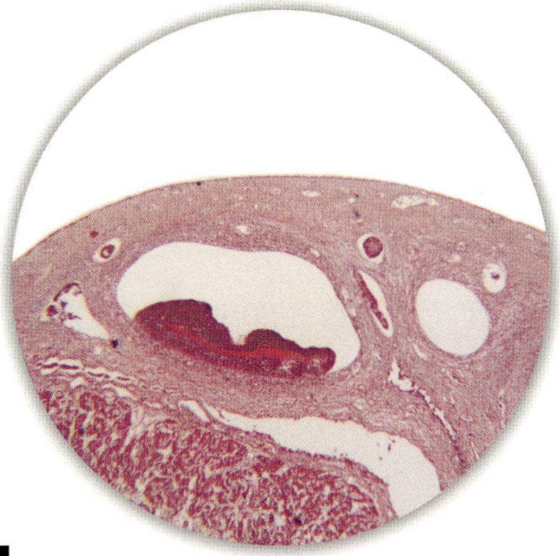

A

58. Fallopian tube (TS) (Fig. 22.4A)

- Highly folded mucosa
- Mucosa lined by simple ciliated columnar epithelium
- Inner circular and outer longitudinal muscle coat.

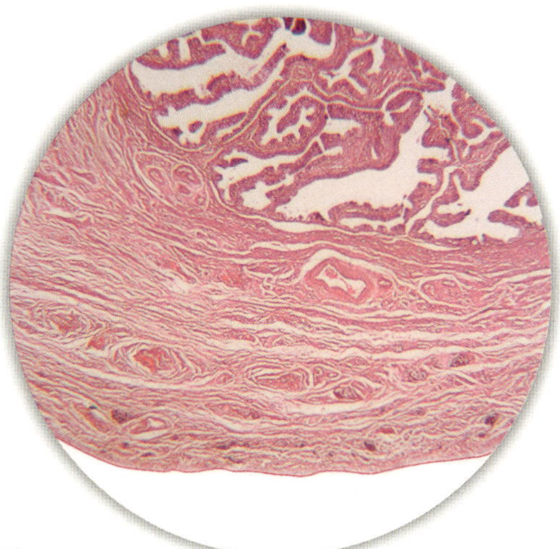

A

59. Uterus (Proliferative phase) (Fig. 22.5A)

- Endometrium lined by simple columnar epithelium
- Lamina propria containing uterine glands
- Thick myometrium with numerous blood vessels.

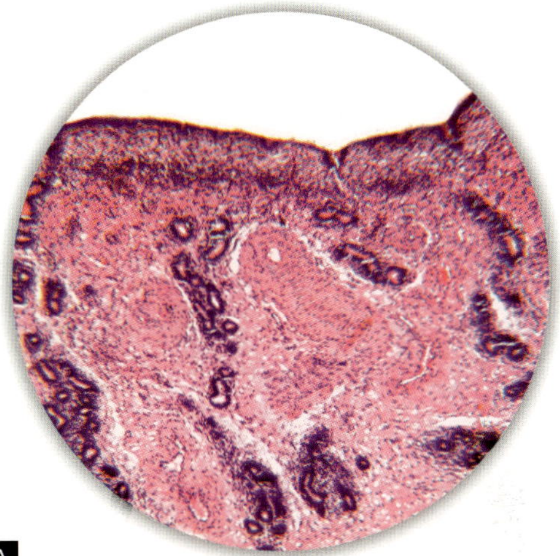

A

60. Cerebrum (Fig. 23.2A)

- Outer pia mater
- Six layered cells are present
- Inner and outer bands of Baillarger are visible.

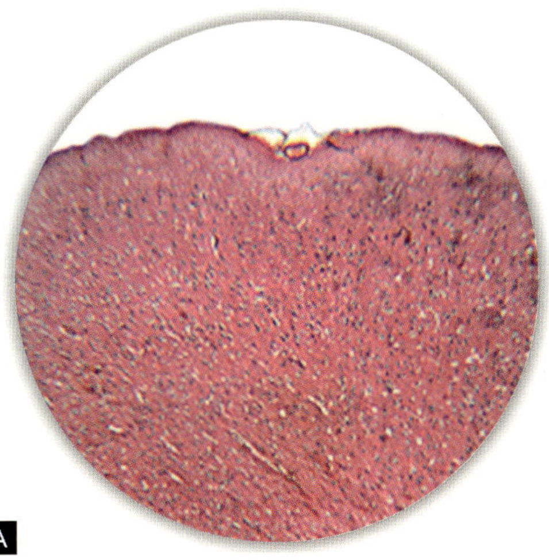

A

61. Cerebellum (Fig. 23.3A)

- Outer molecular layer
- Middle Purkinje cell layer
- Inner granular layer.

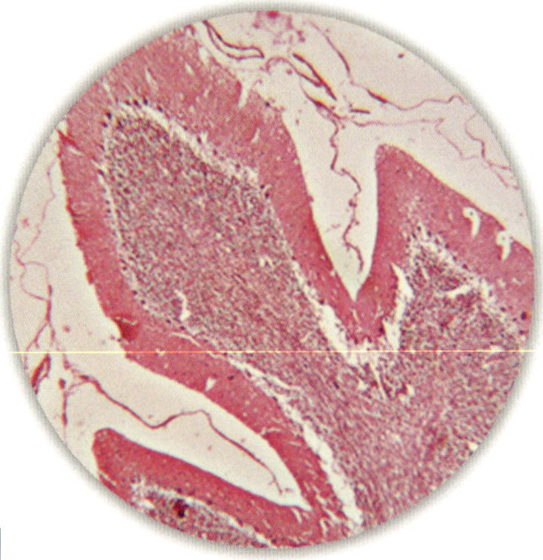

A

62. Spinal cord (Fig. 23.4)

- Outer white matter
- Inner H-shaped gray matter
- Central canal is present.

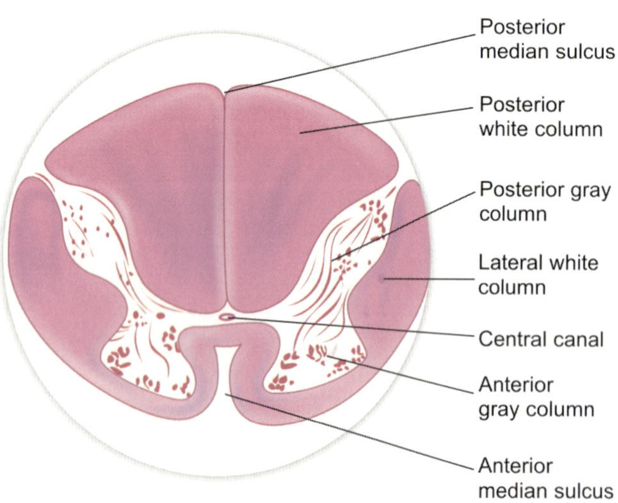

63. Cornea (Fig. 24.1A)

- Outer stratified squamous non-keratinized epithelium
- Intermediate stroma
- Inner endothelial lining.

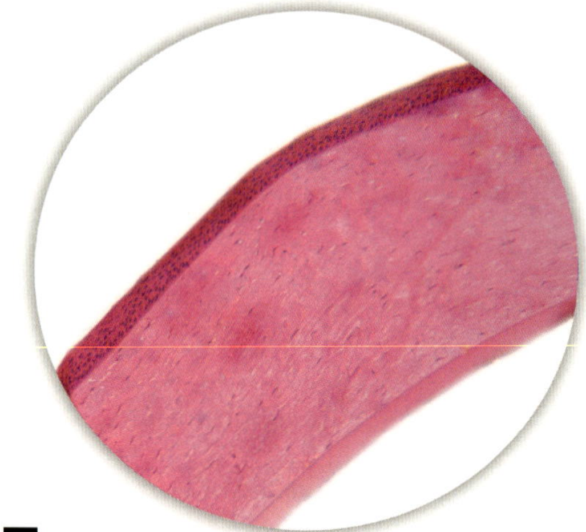

A

64. Eyeball (Retina) (Fig. 24.2A)

- Outermost pigment cell layer
- Middle plexiform and nuclear layer
- Innermost internal limiting membrane.

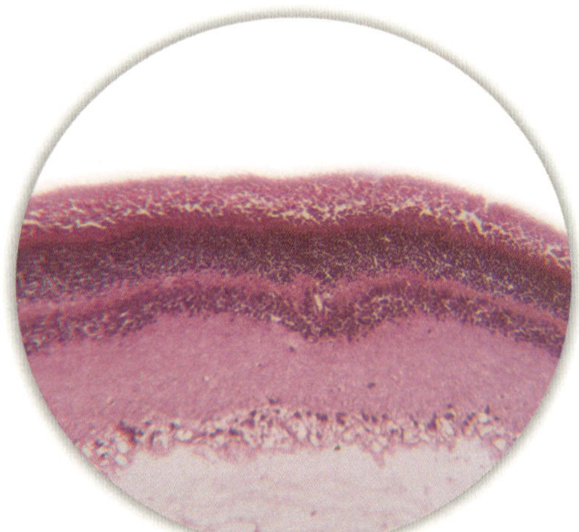

A

65. Tooth (LS) (Fig. 13.1)

- Outermost enamel
- Prominent dentin with dentinal tubules
- Dental pulp containing blood vessels and nerve fibers in it.

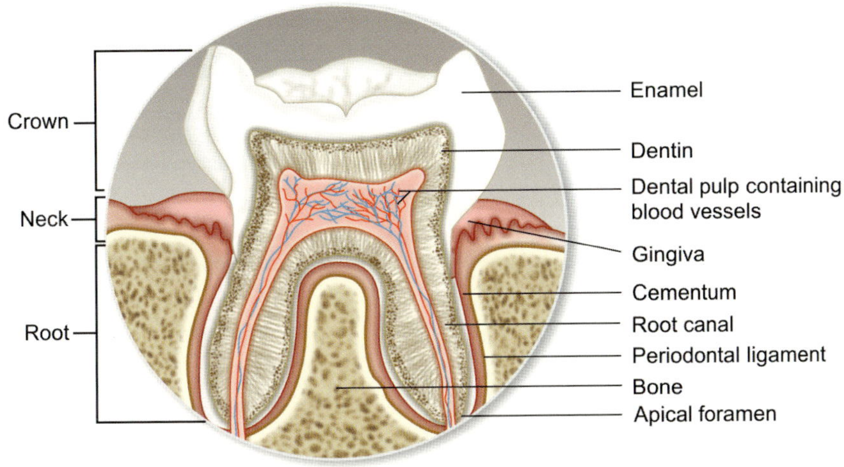

66. Uterus (Secretory phase) (Fig. 22.6)

- Thick endometrium lined by simple columnar epithelium
- Lamina propria containing tortuous glands and coiled arteries
- Myometrium with numerous blood vessels.

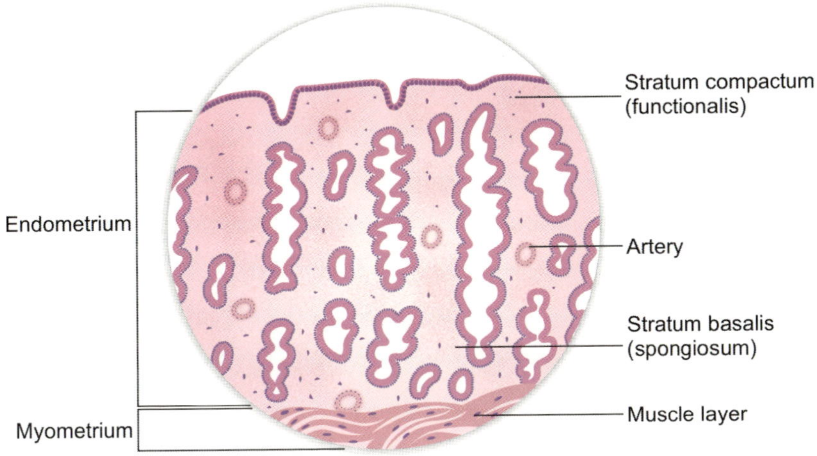

67. Mammary gland (Lactating) (Fig. 22.7)

- Numerous prominent acinar lobules
- Acinar lobules lined by simple columnar epithelium
- Minimal connective tissue with duct system.

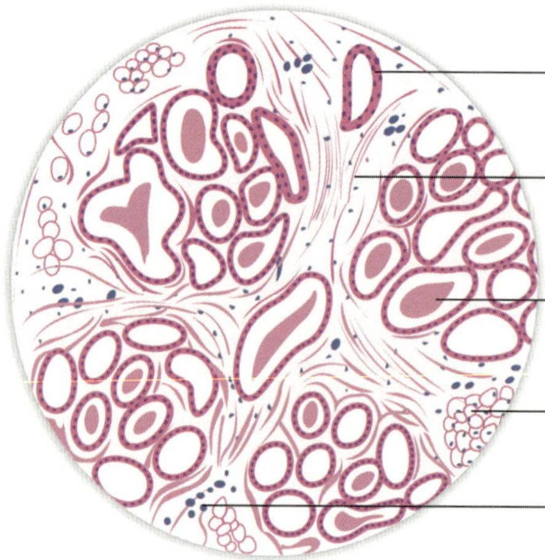

68. Umbilical cord (Fig. 22.8)

- Two umbilical arteries
- One umbilical vein
- Wharton's jelly is present.

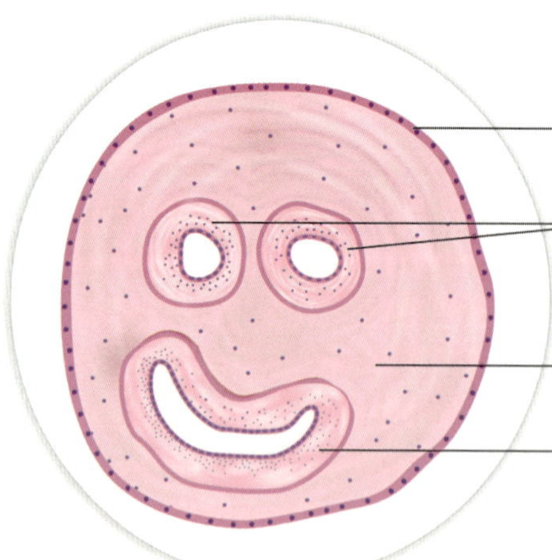

CHAPTER

2 History of Histology

Innumerable of scientists have worked in the field of 'Histology' to explain more about its origin, evolution and advancements with a clear and a better view. Let us consider few great personalities, who tried to build the history of Histology.

ROBERT HOOKE (Fig. 2.1)

Robert Hooke was born in Isle of Wight in the year 1635. His father John Hooke was a curate of Freshwater's Church of All Saints and was expecting his son to join the church soon after his education. But, Robert Hooke was a fascinated person and always wanted to know more and more about the life. And finally his interest about the life made him to discover the **cell**.

When he observed a **piece of cork** under a **micrographia** designed by him, he could realize many small living entities and named it as cell. The word cell comes from Latin **cellule,** which means a small room. Since he compared the cork cells to the small rooms in which monks lived in, hence the name **cell**. This was the first and most valuable discovery, which started building the history of histology.

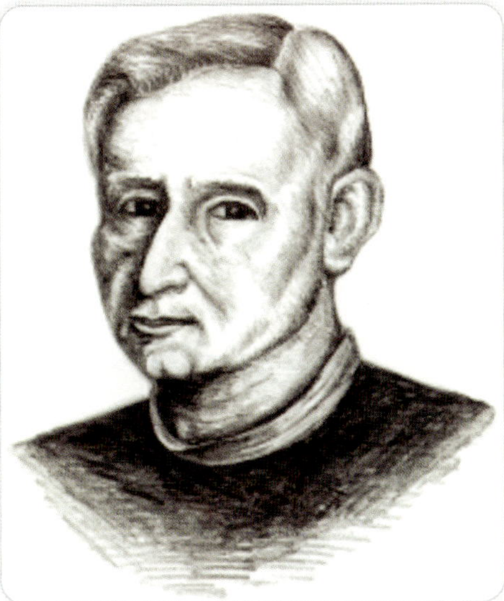

Figure 2.1: Robert Hooke

ANTONIE VAN LEEUWENHOEK (Fig. 2.2)

Antonie was born in Delft on October 24, 1632. His father was a basket maker, seeing him, Antonie started building his career in business as a minor draper (a fabric merchant) and later he also worked as a surveyor, a wine assayer and as a minor city official.

After some time (in 1668), Antonie learned to grind the lenses and designed a simple microscope. He started observing different kinds of objects in it. Even though simple microscope was made up of powerful magnifying lenses, he could visualize the objects 200 times more bigger than its actual size with a better, clearer and brighter images.

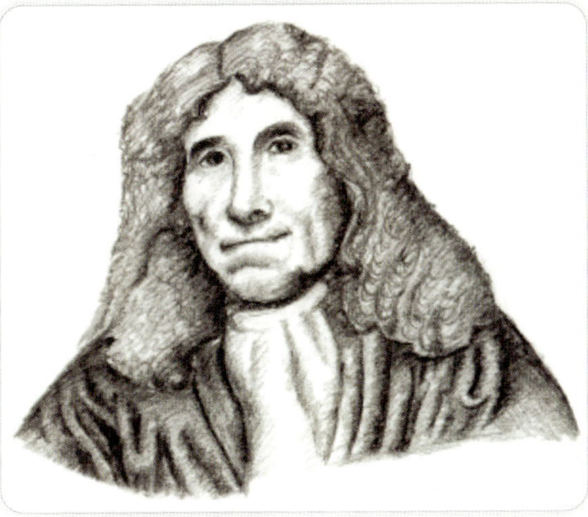

Figure 2.2: Antonie van Leeuwenhoek

According to some people, **"Antonie van Leeuwenhoek was an unlikely scientist."** Since he had no family background in research, received no higher education or university degrees and knew no languages other than his native Dutch, but his skills at grinding lenses, natural eagle's eyesight, light adjustments, great curiosity to observe almost everything which comes to his hands and a special care in describing what he saw, made him enter the Royal Society of London.

Bacteria, blood cells, living sperms, microscopic rotifers and protistas are few of his discoveries and the list of his discoveries go on.

ROBERT BROWN (Fig. 2.3)

Robert Brown was born in Montrose, Scotland on 21st December 1773. He was a famous botanist in Australia during the first half of the 19th century.

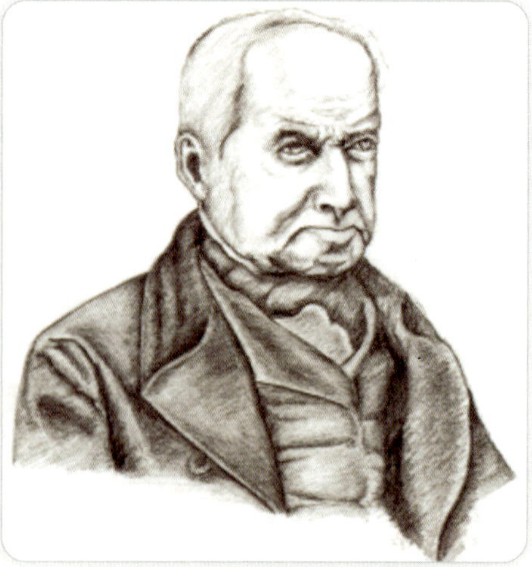

Figure 2.3: Robert Brown

After his medical study at the University of Edinburgh, he was appointed as army surgeon. Later he accepted naturalist post. He also did an intensive botanical research in Australia for three and a half years during which he discovered and coined the term **Nucleus**. He was also a well-recognized person for his **Brownian motion** phenomenon.

MARIE FRANÇOIS XAVIER BICHAT (Fig. 2.4)

Marie François Xavier Bichat was a French anatomist and physiologist born in Thoirette on November 14, 1771. He also worked in the field of mathematics and physical sciences, but ultimately dedicated his life to the study of anatomy and surgery. He did an intensive study in the field of Histology and Pathology. He also coined the term **Tissue**, which means a fabric. He also introduced the concept of "**Diseases attack tissue rather than the whole organ**".

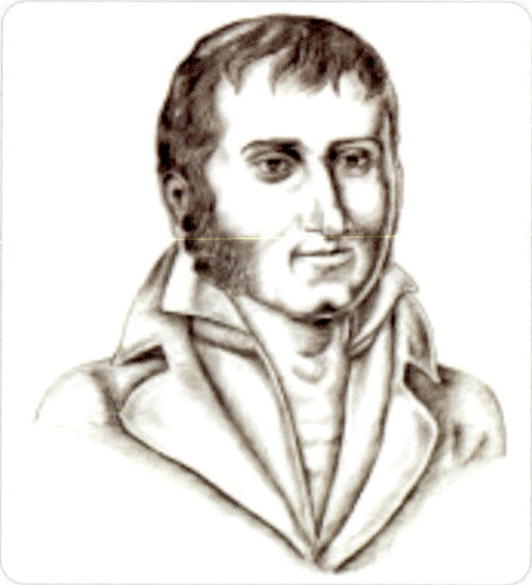

Figure 2.4: Marie François Xavier Bichat

Now he is best remembered as **"The Father of Modern Histology and Pathology"**.

RUDOLF ALBERT VON KÖLLIKER (Fig. 2.5)

Albert von Kölliker was a Swiss anatomist and physiologist born in Zurich, Switzerland on July 6, 1817. He worked in the University of Wuzburg as a professor of Physiology and comparative anatomy.

Kölliker's dedications in the field of Zoology and Embryology are remembered. His discoveries in the field of Histology are innumerable and unlimited. Kölliker demonstrated that **smooth muscle** is made up of distinct units

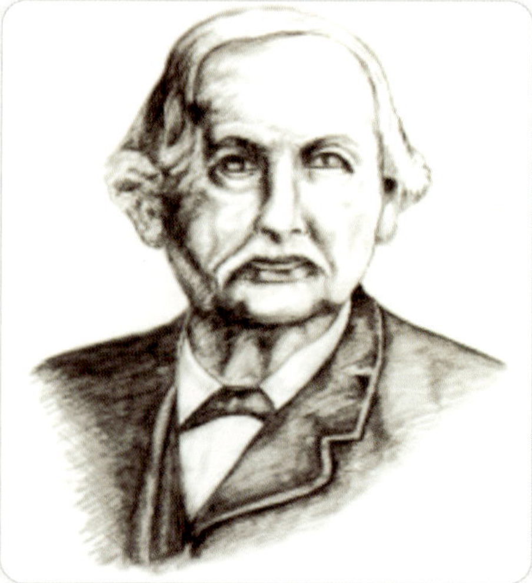

Figure 2.5: Rudolf Albert von Kölliker

of nucleated muscle cells; he also demonstrated the presence of **mitochondria** in the cell.

Skin, bone, teeth, blood vessels, viscera, smooth and striated muscle have been investigated by Kölliker with a special work on Histology of nervous system. **In fact, he was among the first to introduce and improve the hardening, sectioning, staining techniques in Histology**. Finally, Kölliker's work grabbed the Royal Society's attention and made him a part of it in 1860.

THEODOR SCHWANN (Fig. 2.6)

Theodor Schwann was a German physiologist, histologist and cytologist born in Neuss on December 7, 1810. His father was a goldsmith, later a printer.

Schwann's contribution to biology includes the development of **cell theory**, discovery of **Schwann cell**, discovery and study of **pepsin enzyme**, discovery of **organic nature of yeast**, coined the term **Metabolism**, etc.

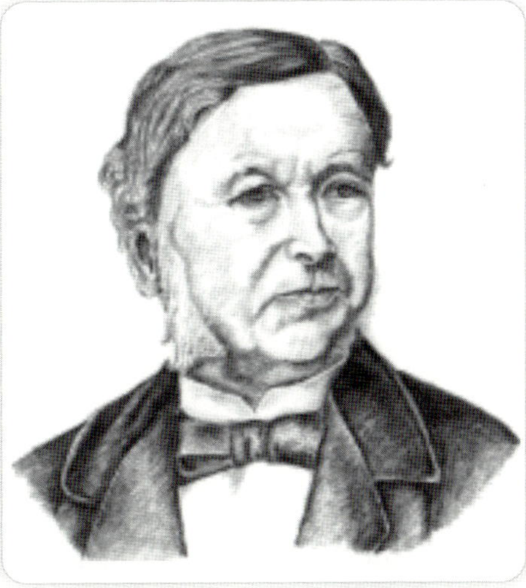

Figure 2.6: Theodor Schwann

He did an intensive study on Histology of peripheral nervous system and he also stained the nerve cells by using silver stains and its compounds, which was popular as **Black reaction**. He died on January 11, 1882.

Chapter 3

General Instructions

- A medical student should enter the histology practical hall with clean and well-ironed medical coat (apron).
- It is mandatory to enter the histology practical hall with practical record book, an observation book and other requirements.
- A medical student should behave decently in the practical class and carry out his/her practical without disturbing other students.
- Each student is responsible for the safety of the microscope given to him/her during the practical classes.
- Remember that the microscope is a delicate and costly instrument. It should be used carefully and wiped clean after using.
- A medical student is not allowed to touch the slides or change the field of the slides, which are kept for the demonstration.
- Histological slides should be handled gently and special care should be taken not to damage the slides.
- Practical record book should be maintained properly and neatly. They must be submitted for inspection to the Professor of Anatomy as and when required.
- Student should get his/her practical record initialed at the conclusion of each class by the lecturer in-charge. This should never be postponed to the next class.
- Students are strictly advised to return the histological slides and the microscope in a good condition before leaving histology practical hall.
- At the conclusion of the course before appearing for the university examination, student should submit the record book on the date duly notified for scrutiny and signature of the staff in-charge and head of the department of anatomy.

The university examination register number should be entered clearly on the practical record book before the final submission.

METHOD OF DRAWING THE FIGURES IN HISTOLOGY

Drawing the diagrams in Histology is an art. A proper knowledge about different cells, their staining characters and a bit of neatness makes the histological diagrams more attractive and meaningful.

A charming figure in the examination always attracts the examiners and helps to fetch more marks.

So, here is a list of tips to make the diagrams more attractive and meaningful.

Hematoxylin and eosin staining is most widely used staining technique in Histology. Hence, knowledge about the staining characters of different cells should guide the use of appropriate colors for the histology figures as given below:

- Nucleus and nucleolus stain blue (hematoxylin).
- Cytoplasm, collagen fibers and muscle cells stain pink (eosin).
- A serous cell stains pink to bright red whereas a mucus cell stains faint blue to purple.

  Note: Histology of the bone, tooth and nerve should be drawn only with the help of normal lead (HB) pencils.
- It is better to draw the diagrams first in the observation book and then in the practical record book, so that you can correct the mistakes made in the observation book and thus prepare accurate and good figures in the practical record book.

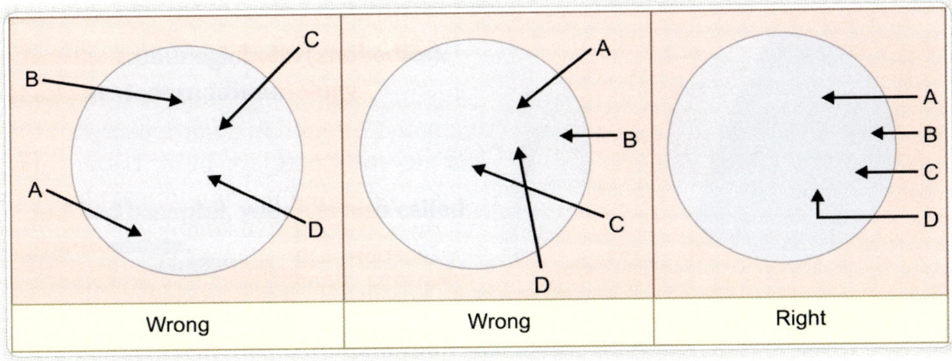

Figure 3.1: Method of labeling diagrams

- Always develop a habit of drawing a circle and writing the diagrams within it, see to it that the figure should not come out of the circle's margin.
- It is better to keep a compass and a small size metallic bangle or kada for drawing the circle.
- Often students complain that hematoxylin and eosin pencils are quite delicate compared to normal pencils and they cannot be sharpened. So, it is better to use a blade to make the pencils sharp.

  Note: **"Neat and attractive figures can be drawn only with nicely sharpened pencils".**
- Use a good quality eraser so that it would not leave behind any marks even after erasing the mistakes. Do not be rough, while erasing, otherwise the paper may tear, which gives a bad impression.
- Always try to label the diagrams on one side (usually on the right side). It prevents confusion in the identification of different structures. Make sure that the figure and its beauty is not destroyed while labeling (Fig. 3.1).
- Always use a transparent ruler for labeling the diagrams. Usually, the students label the diagrams without using the scale and the lines drawn look very funny!

Even though the tips described above may sound funny, but these are the common mistakes committed by students, while drawing the histological diagrams. Hence, accurate and meaningful figures are drawn only when such silly mistakes are corrected!

REQUIREMENTS IN HISTOLOGY

- A practical record book.
- An observation book.
- Hematoxylin and eosin pencils.
- A simple lead pencil, eraser, sharpener, blade and a transparent scale (15 cm) (Fig. 3.2).

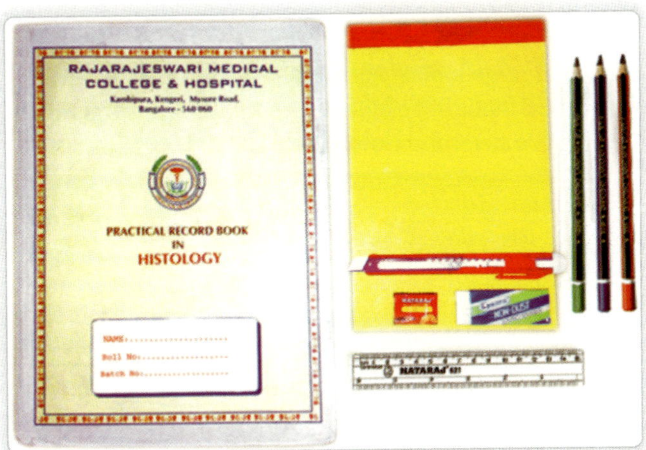

Figure 3.2: Requirements in histology

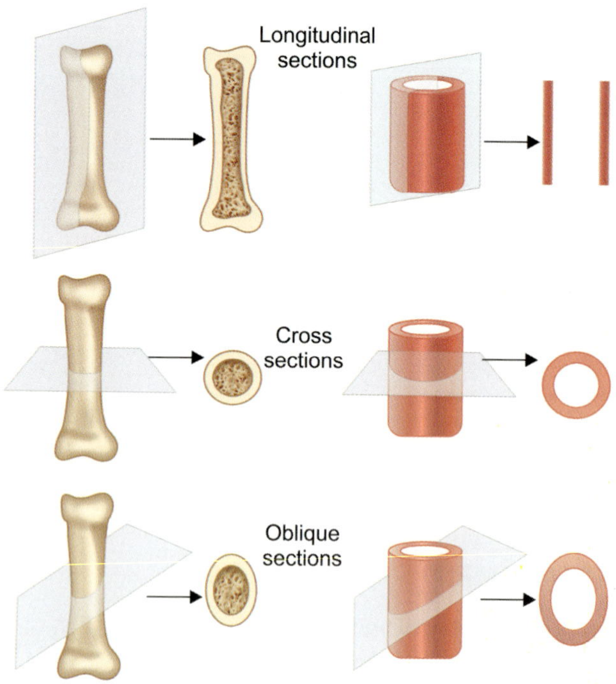

Figure 3.3: Different planes of sections in histology

DIFFERENT PLANES OF SECTIONS IN HISTOLOGY

Before staining any slide, first the tissue or organ will be cut or sectioned in a particular plane so that the cells and other structures are more better appreciated (Fig. 3.3). Following are the commonest planes used to section the tissues/organs in histology. Please observe the differences among different planes of sections:

- Longitudinal section (LS).
- Transverse section (TS) or cross section.
- Oblique section.

Chapter

4 Study of Microscope

Microscope is an amazing device in the history of science, which helped a lot in elaborating the fields of Histology, Pathology, Microbiology, Genetics and Forensic medicine. Microscope is a Greek term, which means **a device used to look at smaller objects** (micro; small, skopein; to examine).

TYPES OF MICROSCOPES

Different types of microscopes are:

- **Simple microscope:** It is a microscope with single magnifying lens.
- **Compound microscope:** A microscope having two or more objective lenses with different magnifications with single eyepiece.
- **Binocular microscope:** It is a microscope having two eye pieces with two or more objective lenses.
- **Dark field microscope:** Here reflected light rays are used to view the microscopic objects.
- **Electron microscope:** Here a beam of electrons are used to view the microscopic objects.
- **Light microscope:** It is an ordinary microscope in which visible light is used to view the microscopic objects.

Other types of microscope are:

- Phase contrast microscope.
- Operating microscope.
- Polarization microscope.
- Scanning electron microscope.
- Stereoscopic microscope.
- Ultraviolet microscope.
- X-ray microscope.
- Slit-lamp microscope, etc.

COMPONENTS OF COMPOUND MICROSCOPE

A schematic diagram of a compound microscope and its parts are as shown in Figure 4.1 and it can be described under following headings:

- **Support system.**
- **Illumination system.**
- **Magnification system.**
- **Adjustment system.**

Support System

Support system is the framework of the microscope, which holds the different parts together for a better function. Following are the different parts of the supporting system.

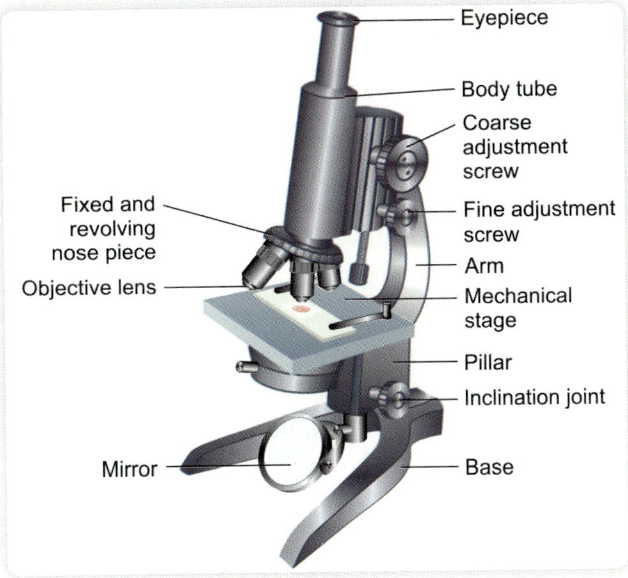

Figure 4.1: Compound microscope

Base: It is a horse shoe-shaped structure, which bears the entire weight of the microscope on it. It also gives good stability to the microscope.

Pillars: These are the connecting structures, which connect the base to the handle of the microscope.

Arm (Handle): It is a C-shaped structure, which forms a bridge between mechanical stage and body tube. With the help of the arm one can easily carry and tilt the microscope at a desirable level.

Body tube: It is a cylindrical-shaped structure, which carries the light from mirror to eye piece.

Mechanical stage: It is a fixed horizontal platform on which the glass slide is placed. It consists of central aperture through which light enters the slide and a pair of clips, which hold the glass slide in a fixed position. Mechanical stage is also provided with a pair of screws, which help in movement of glass slide in forward, backward and transverse direction.

Nose piece: It is a round plate like structure, which consists of upper fixed nose piece and lower revolving nose piece. The upper fixed nose piece connects with the body tube where as the lower revolving nose piece bears the objective lenses of varying magnifying powers.

Illumination System

Illumination system is the light system of the microscope, which provides an adequate light adjustment for the better visualization of the smaller objects. It consists of following parts.

Light source: It helps in visualization of objects with greater details. It is of two types, external and internal. The **external light source** is the source of light either sunlight or electric lamps and the **internal light source** is the source of light of an electrical lamp, which is fitted to the microscope during its design. Most of the current microscopes in the market are said to be internal light source fitted microscopes.

Mirror: It is seen at the base of the microscope just below the condenser. It has two surfaces, plane mirror surface, which is used for oil immersion objectives and concave surface, which is used for the low and high power objectives.

Condenser: As the name itself indicates it helps in condensing the light rays, which are reflected from mirror onto the object. It is important to note that the condenser should be fixed at its lowest level when a low power objective is used. It is to be raised optimally, while using high power objective and it is to be raised fully, when oil immersion objective is used.

Iris diaphragm: It is found just below the condenser, which helps in controlling the number of light rays entering the condenser. An iris diaphragm works very much similar to that of the iris of the eye, hence the name.

Magnification System

Magnification system is an important system of any microscope, which is responsible for the magnification of the micro-objects. It consists of eye piece and objectives. **Please note that the total magnification of any microscope is the sum of magnification of eye piece and the objective chosen.**

Eye piece: It is a lens fitted on top of the body tube by which an examiner examines the objects in microscope. The usual magnification of the eye piece is 10X, however eye piece with magnification power of 8X, 5X and 2X are also used in practice. A microscope with one eye piece is called **monocular microscope,** where as a microscope with two eye pieces is called **binocular microscope.**

Objectives: These are lenses with different magnification powers, which are fitted on to the revolving nose piece and they are:

- Low power objective (10X).
- High power objective (40X).
- Oil immersion objective (100X).

Low power objective: It is an objective lens with magnification power of 10X. It is usually used for identification and scanning the object. Low power objective helps in having an overview of the object (slide).

Note: In examination most of the slides for spotters will be focused under low power objective.

High power objective: It is an objective lens with magnification power of 40X. It is usually used for the detailed study of the slide.

Oil immersion objective: It is an objective with magnification of 100X. It is usually used for studying the morphology of the cells. In this objective immersion oil is used to form a close contact between the objective and the slide. The most commonly used immersion oils are **cedar wood oil** and **castor oil.**

Magnification Power

It is important to understand that the magnification power of a lens is the ability of the lens to magnify the object. If the magnification power of a lens (low power objective) is 10X, then it means that under low power objective cells appear 10 times bigger than the actual size.

Total magnification power of a microscope = Magnification of eye piece + Magnification of the objective

Keeping the magnification power of eyepiece (10X) stable and changing the objective lenses then the magnification power of a microscope with low objective microscope will be,

$$10X \times 10X = 100X$$

Adjustment System

Following are the two different adjustment systems used in the microscope.

Coarse adjustment: These are the bigger screws, which are mounted at the top of the handle and they help in coarse adjustment. Here both the screws are interconnected, hence when one screw is rotated then the opposite screw rotates automatically.

Fine adjustment: These are the smaller screws, which are in the handle just below the coarse adjustment screws and they help in fine adjustment, and focusing of the object for a better view.

EXAMINATION OF SLIDE

Following are the simple instructions to examine the slides:

- Take the microscope to a moderately illuminated day light area (Fig. 4.2).
- Gently wipe the eye piece and plane mirror with a piece of cotton to get a bright and good illumination.

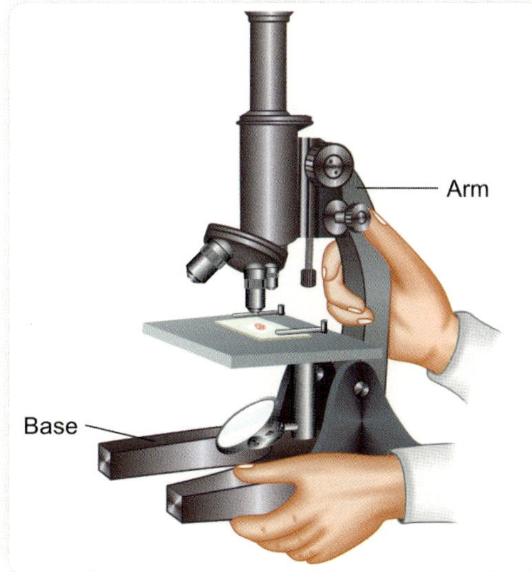

Figure 4.2: Right method of holding the microscope

- Adjust the plain mirror and condenser in such a way that a clear bright circle of light is seen through the eye piece.
- Place the slide on mechanical stage and fix the slide with protective clips to ensure the safety of slide.
- Examine the slide under low magnification (10X) first and then switch on to high magnification (40X) to view the slide in detail.
- In case of oil immersion microscope, place a drop of cedar wood oil or castor oil on the slide and focus the slide by using oil immersion objective (100X).

Note: Do not forget to clean the objective lens, eye piece and mirror at the end of each practical class (especially, if oil immersion objective is used).

SECTION 2

General Histology

CHAPTER

5 Epithelial Tissue

INTRODUCTION

- Epithelial tissue is the most commonly seen tissue in the body, which lines the internal, external and visceral organs
- It was first described as the layer of cells covering the nipple, hence named as epithelium. (epi: upon, thallus: nipple).

CHARACTERISTIC FEATURES

- Epithelial tissue is derived from all the three germ layers of the developing embryo, i.e. ectoderm, endoderm and mesoderm.
- The cells are usually flattened, cuboidal or columnar in shape.
- The cells are either single layered or multilayered.
- In single-layered cells, all the cells are resting on the basement membrane whereas in a multilayered cells only the basal layer cells are resting on the basement membrane.
- The cells are compactly arranged thus there is little or no intercellular space and matrix.
- The epithelial cells are arranged in the form of a continuous sheet or layer.
- Epithelial cells are **avascular** in nature, i.e. they do not have direct blood supply.
- Epithelial tissue has got the high capacity of regeneration, i.e. whenever there is injury or discontinuity in the cell layer, they actively multiply and fill up the gap.

Basement Membrane

- Basement membrane is a thin layer of connective tissue on which the epithelial cells rest.
- It is found just beneath the epithelial cells as a minute, indistinct, narrow streak or line.
- It is made up of glycoproteins and heteropolysaccharides.

Functions

- Basement membrane provides the site for adhesion of epithelial cells.
- Acts as a barrier to the diffusion of molecules.
- Supplies the nutrients and gases to the epithelial cells and also transfers the metabolic waste products and CO_2 from the epithelial cells.

CLASSIFICATION

- Epithelial tissue is mainly classified as **unilayered and multilayered** based on the number of layers of cells present. And they are further classified into many types based on the shape of the cells as follows (Fig. 5.1).
- There is one more type of epithelium called **pseudostratified epithelium** where the cells are single layered, but give the appearance of a multilayered epithelium. For example, pseudostratified columnar epithelium seen in the auditory tube and male urethra.

Simple Squamous Epithelium (Fig. 5.2)

Introduction

- Simple squamous epithelium is the simplest form of epithelial tissue
- As the cells are arranged compactly without any intercellular spaces like the tiles of the floor, hence it is also called **pavement epithelium**.

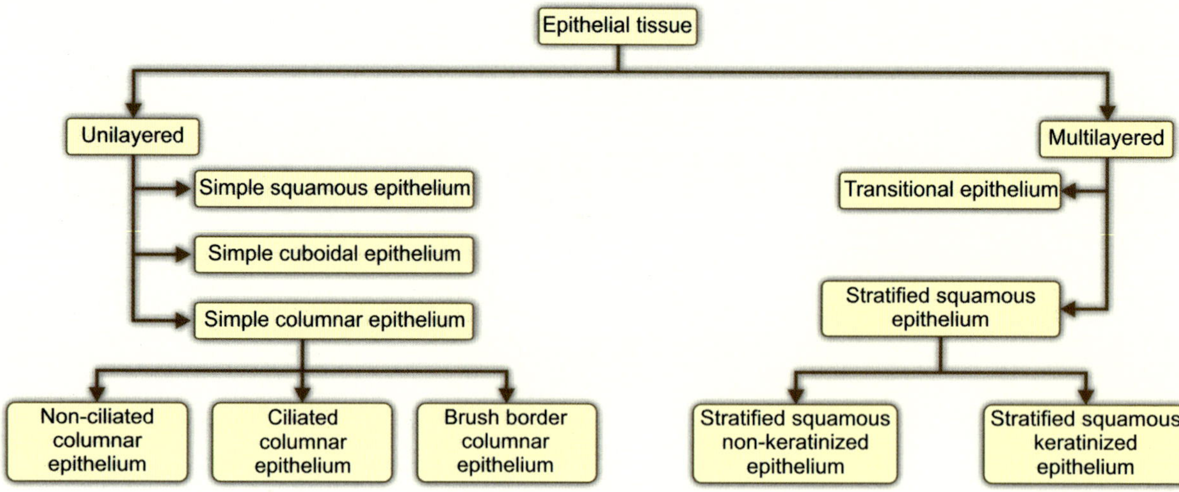

Figure 5.1: Classification of epithelial tissue

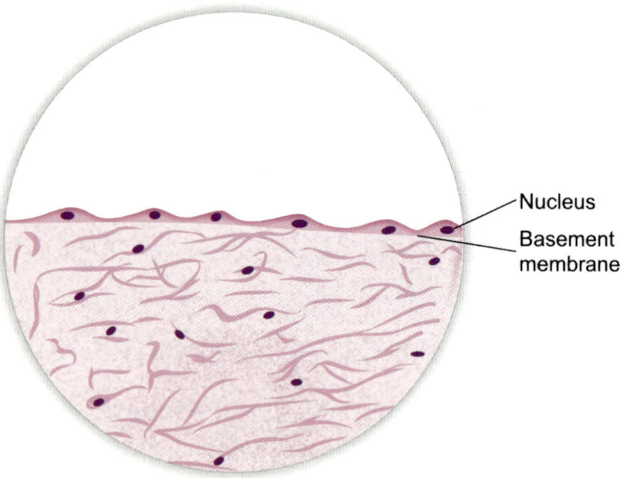

Figure 5.2: Simple squamous epithelium

Cell Structure

- The cells are flat, polygonal or isodiametric or irregular in shape. Typically, they contain scanty cytoplasm with a prominent round to oval nucleus at the centre giving rise to a bulged appearance at the center of the cell.
- All the cells are single layered and compactly arranged without any intercellular space and are held together by the **tight junction.** Here, all the cells are resting on the basement membrane.

Different Forms

- **Endothelium:** Seen as the inner lining of blood vessels and lymphatics.
- **Mesothelium:** Found in the pleura, peritoneum, pericardium and synovial membrane.
- **Endocardium:** Found in the inner wall of the heart.

Occurrence

Alveoli of lungs, inner lining of blood vessels and lymphatics, lining of body cavities (peritoneum, pericardium and pleura) endocardium of heart, parietal layer of Bowman's capsule, thin segment of renal tubules and various parts of internal ear.

Functions

- Protective in function.
- **Antithrombotic** in nature.
- Exchange of respiratory gases takes place in the alveoli of lungs.
- Passive transport of fluid takes place in the pleura and peritoneum, etc.

Simple Cuboidal Epithelium (Fig. 5.3)

Cell Structure

- The cells are cube like with equal height and breadth. The nucleus is round and is placed at the center of the cell with moderate cytoplasm.
- The cells are single layered and compactly arranged without any intercellular space. All the cells here rest on the basement membrane.

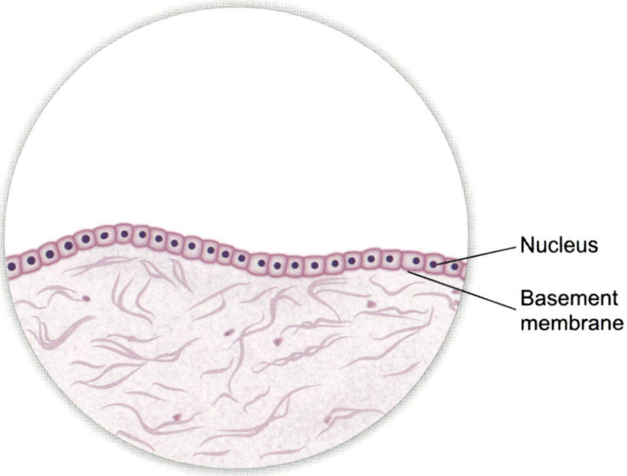

Figure 5.3: Simple cuboidal epithelium

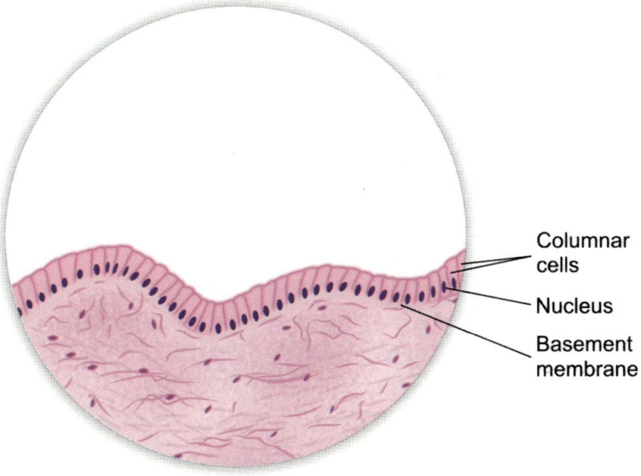

Figure 5.4: Simple columnar epithelium

Occurrence

Follicles of thyroid gland, in the small ducts of glands, on the surface of the ovary (germinal epithelium), choroid plexus, pigmented layer of retina, inner surface of lens and kidney tubules.

Function

Cells are mainly secretary and protective in function.

Simple Columnar Epithelium (Fig. 5.4)

Cell Structure

- Cells are tall, pillar like from the side view (vertical section) and polygonal in shape when viewed horizontally.
- A typical cell is tall, pillar like with a nucleus toward the base of the cell. The cytoplasm of the cell is either clear or contains granules or droplets of secretary materials, which are more around the base of the cell. They have an abundant amount of **Golgi apparatus** in the cell.
- Some of the cells are modified to secrete mucus and they acquire a characteristic shape of a wine glass. Hence, called **goblet cells** and in such cells the mucus is present toward the apex of the cell.
- The cells are single layered and compactly arranged without intercellular space and all the cells here rest on the basement membrane.

Different Forms

- **Simple non-ciliated columnar epithelium:** Here, the surface of columnar cells does not show any specialization and it does not bear either microvilli or cilia.
- **Ciliated columnar epithelium**: Here, the surface of the columnar cells bear small hair-like structures called cilia. The non-motile cilia are called **steriocilia.**
- **Brush border columnar epithelium:** Here, the surface of columnar cells bear small minute finger-like projections called **microvilli** (Table 5.1).

Table 5.1: Differences between cilia and microvilli

Cilia	Microvilli
These are the small hair-like projections arising from the cell surface	These are the minute finger like projections from the cell surface
They are long, elongated and loosely arranged and packed	They are small, short and closely packed
Cilia are motile	Microvilli are non-motile
Rich in microtubules	Rich in microfilaments
Seen even under light microscope	Seen under electron microscope only

Occurrence

- Simple non-ciliated columnar epithelium is seen in the inner lining of gallbladder, stomach, small intestine and colon.

- Ciliated columnar epithelium is seen in most of the respiratory tract (except pharynx and vocal folds). The uterus, uterine tube, efferent ductules of testes, few parts of middle ear and auditory tube.
- Brush border columnar epithelium is seen in proximal convoluted tubule of the nephrons in kidney.

Functions

- Simple non-ciliated columnar epithelium is absorptive in function and they absorb the digested food particles in the small and large intestine.
- It is also secretary in function and secretes mucus, which protects the inner wall of stomach from acid secretions.
- Ciliated columnar epithelium performs the **ciliary action** by which they trap the dust, helping in the movement of the dust and other foreign particles in same direction (upwards).
- Brush border columnar epithelial cells present in the renal tubules help in the absorption of nutrients and fluid from the filtrate, which passes through the renal tubule.

Transitional Epithelium (Figs 5.5A and B)

Introduction

- Transitional epithelium is a multilayered epithelium, which is four to six cell layers thick
- The epithelium is called **transitional epithelium,** because its layers are transitory or variable with different stages of distention. Since, the transitional epithelium is mainly found in the urinary tract, it is also named as **urothelium**.

Cell Structure

Cells are multilayered and compactly arranged without the intercellular space. Here, the basal cells are columnar or cuboidal in shape and are resting on the basement membrane. The middle layer of cells are either polyhedral or pear-shaped in nature and the outermost layer of cells are either balloon or umbrella shaped hence, the outermost layer of cells are also called **umbrella cells**.

Occurrence

Renal pelvis, calyces, ureter, urinary bladder and a small part of urethra.

Functions

- It increases the capacity of the urine storage in the bladder by stretching without getting cut and by reducing in number of layers.
- Since the outermost layer cells (umbrella cells) are compactly arranged, which act as urine proof and prevent the reabsorption of waste toxic products of urine back to the tissues and blood.

Stratified Squamous Epithelium

Cell Structure

- In this, the cells are multilayered and compactly arranged without any intercellular space.

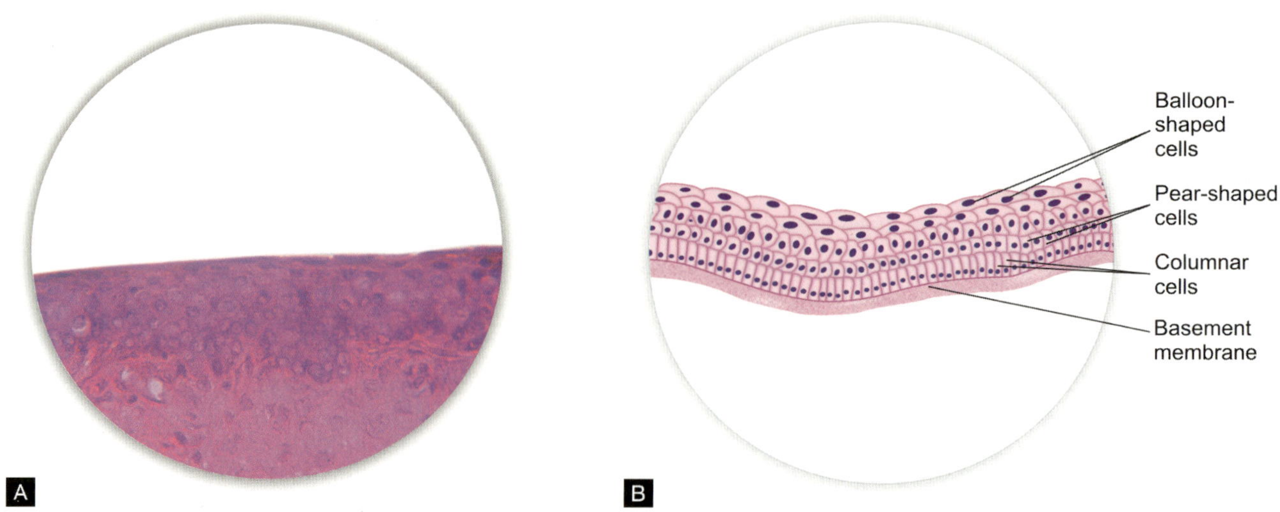

Figures 5.5A and B: Transitional epithelium. **A.** Photograph; **B.** Diagrammatic representation.

- Here, the basal cells are columnar in shape and are resting on the basement membrane, the cells in the middle layer are either cuboidal or polyhedral in shape. As we pass through the peripheral surface of epithelium, the cells become more flat and large.
- Here, the basal cells are the most active cells whereas the peripheral cells are degenerating or dead cells.

Types

1. **Stratified squamous non-keratinized epithelium.**
2. **Stratified squamous keratinized epithelium.**

Stratified squamous non-keratinized epithelium (Figs 5.6A and B)

Introduction

- Stratified squamous non-keratinized epithelium is seen where the surface of the epithelium remains moist and there is no layer of keratin deposit.

Occurrence

Oral cavity, esophagus, tongue, vagina, cornea and upper half of anal canal.

Stratified squamous keratinized epithelium (Figs 5.7A and B)

- This type of epithelium is seen where the surface of the body is dry and there is an outermost layer of keratin deposit.
- This type of epithelium usually contains the appendages of the skin (hair, sweat glands and sebaceous glands).

Occurrence

Sole of the foot and hand, epidermis of the skin, lower half of the anal canal.

Functions

- The epithelium of the skin protects the underlying tissues from being dried out from temperature variations such as heat, cold, etc.
- The epithelial lining of the esophagus withstands wear and tear as the food passes through it.
- **Keratin,** a sulfur containing protein present on the skin acts as an antibacterial, thus providing protection from the microorganisms and their infections.

Pseudostratified Columnar Epithelial Tissue (Figs 5.8A and B)

Pseudostratified columnar epithelium is a type of epithelium where the cells are single layered, but they give an appearance of multilayered epithelium.

Cell Structure

- Cells are single layered and are compactly arranged without the intercellular space, here all the cells are resting on the basement membrane.
- The cells are columnar in shape, but some cells are broader near the base and others near the apex and the nuclei lie in the border part of each cell. Thus, it gives an impression of multilayered nuclei, which is seen in the multilayered epithelial tissue. Hence, to distinguish this kind of epithelium from the true stratified epithelium, it is named as **pseudostratified columnar epithelium**. If the cells bear cilia, then it is called **pseudostratified ciliated columnar epithelium**.

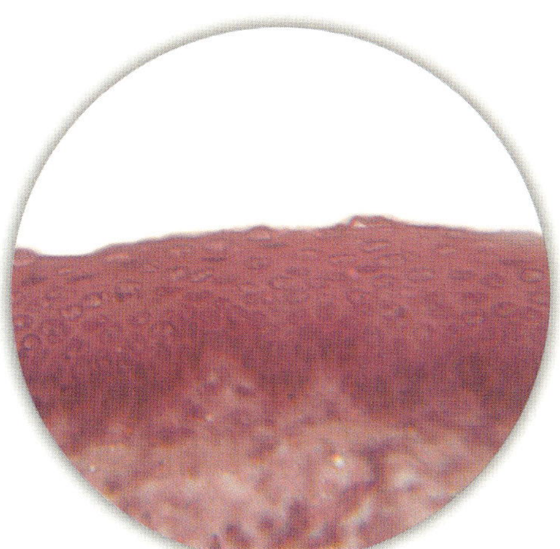

A

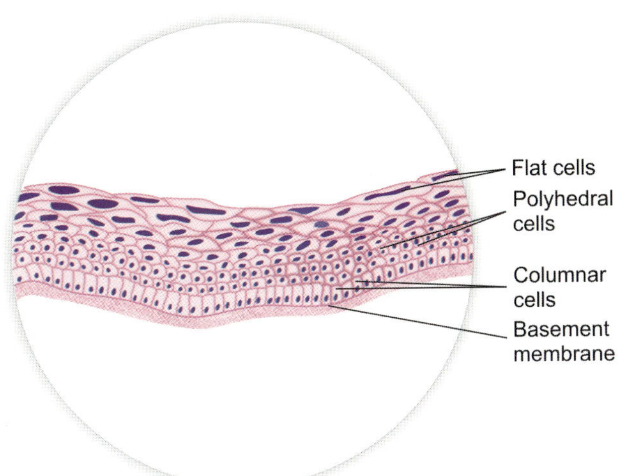

B

Figures 5.6A and B: Stratified squamous non-keratinized epithelium. **A.** Photograph; **B.** Diagrammatic representation.

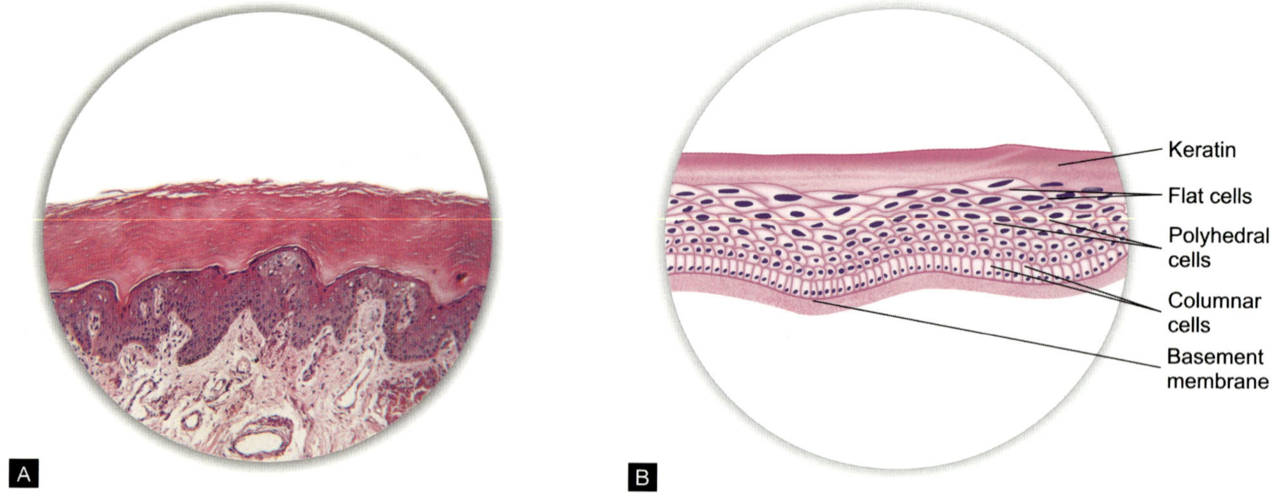

Figures 5.7A and B: Stratified squamous keratinized epithelium. **A.** Photograph; **B.** Diagrammatic representation.

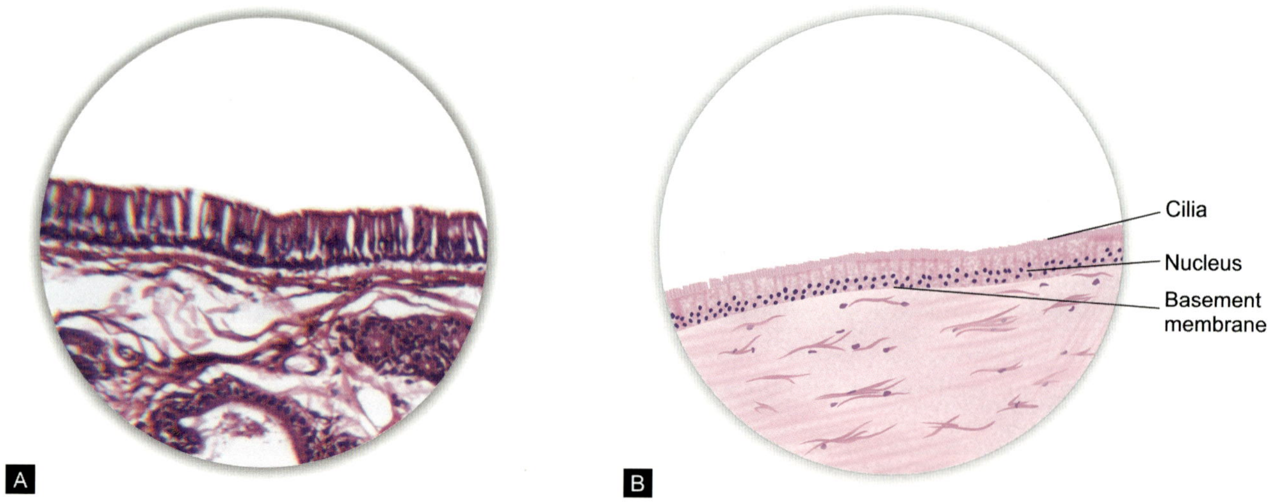

Figures 5.8A and B: Pseudostratified ciliated columnar epithelium. **A.** Photograph; **B.** Diagrammatic representation.

Occurrence

- Pseudostratified columnar epithelium is seen in male urethra, some parts of auditory tube and the ductus deferens.
- Pseudostratified ciliated columnar epithelium is seen in the nasal cavity, trachea and bronchi.

Functions

- Protective in function.
- Moistens the air.
- Warms the air.
- Sterilizes the air.
- Cilia of the cells trap the dust and show the **ciliary reflex**.
- Mucus produced by the cells helps in removing foreign particles from the respiratory tract.

Discussions

- What do you mean by the word epithelium?
- What are the characteristic features of epithelial tissue?
- Name the germ layer, which gives rise to epithelial tissue.
- Classify the epithelial tissue.
- What is basement membrane?

- Where do you see?
  - Simple squamous epithelium.
  - Simple cuboidal epithelium.
  - Simple columnar epithelium.
  - Transitional epithelium.
  - Pseudostratified ciliated columnar epithelium.
  - Stratified squamous keratinized epithelium.
  - Stratified squamous non-keratinized epithelium?
- What are the functions of epithelial tissue?
- List the differences between cilia and microvilli.
- What is the significance of keratin?
- What is the other name for transitional epithelium? Why is it called so?
- Differentiate stratified squamous non-keratinized epithelium from stratified squamous keratinized epithelium.
- What is endothelium and mesothelium?
- Why is the simple squamous epithelium also called pavement epithelium?
- What are goblet cells? What do they secrete?
- Where do you see pseudostratified columnar epithelial tissue? How is it different from other types of epithelial tissue?

Chapter

6 Connective Tissue

INTRODUCTION

Connective tissue is a type of tissue, which provides structural and metabolic support to other tissues and organs. They play an important role in fat storage, defense mechanism and tissue repair.

CHARACTERISTIC FEATURES

- Connective tissue is mesodermal in origin. Connective tissue in an undifferentiated form is called **mesenchyme.**
- An important feature of the connective tissue is the presence of extracellular material called **matrix**, which is secreted by the connective tissue cells.
- Unlike the epithelial tissue, here the cells are not arranged compactly, there is a wide gap between the cells of the connective tissue and the intercellular space is filled by the **extra-cellular matrix.**
- Cells of the connective tissue vary in their size, shape, structure and function.
- In general any connective tissue is rich in fibers, which are of different types and are produced by fibroblasts.

CLASSIFICATION

Connective tissue is mainly classified into two types:

- Specialized connective tissue.
- Connective tissue proper.

Further classification of the connective tissue is as shown in the Figure 6.1.

Note: Blood and lymph are also part of connective tissue and are considered as **fluid connective tissue**.

CONSTITUENTS

- Connective tissue is mainly made up of two parts, i.e. the cellular part and extracellular matrix.
- Cellular part includes different types of cells whereas the extracellular matrix consisting of fibers and ground substance.
- A schematic representation of the constituent of the connective tissue is as shown in the Figure 6.2.

CELLS OF THE CONNECTIVE TISSUE

Fibroblast (Fig. 6.3)

- These are the most abundant type of cells found in connective tissue.
- An active form of cell is known as **fibroblast,** when it becomes old and inactive it is referred as **fibrocyte.**
- A fibroblast is an immature spindle or irregular-shaped cell with an oval nucleus at the center.
- The cytoplasm is more basophilic, rich in rough endoplasmic reticulum and Golgi complex.
- It is said to be a **non-motile (fixed) cell** and always seen in contact with the collagen fibers.

Functions

- Responsible for the production of fibers (collagen, elastic and reticular fibers).
- It secretes the extracellular matrix of the connective tissue.

Adipocytes (Fig. 6.4)

- These are also called **fat cells** or **lipocytes** and aggregation of such cells forms the **adipose tissue.**
- An adipocyte is a round or oval-shaped cell with peripherally pushed flat nucleus.
- Here, whole of the cell is filled with fat globule, thus the cytoplasm of the cell appears as a thin rim around the fat globule, thus forming a **signet ring appearance.**

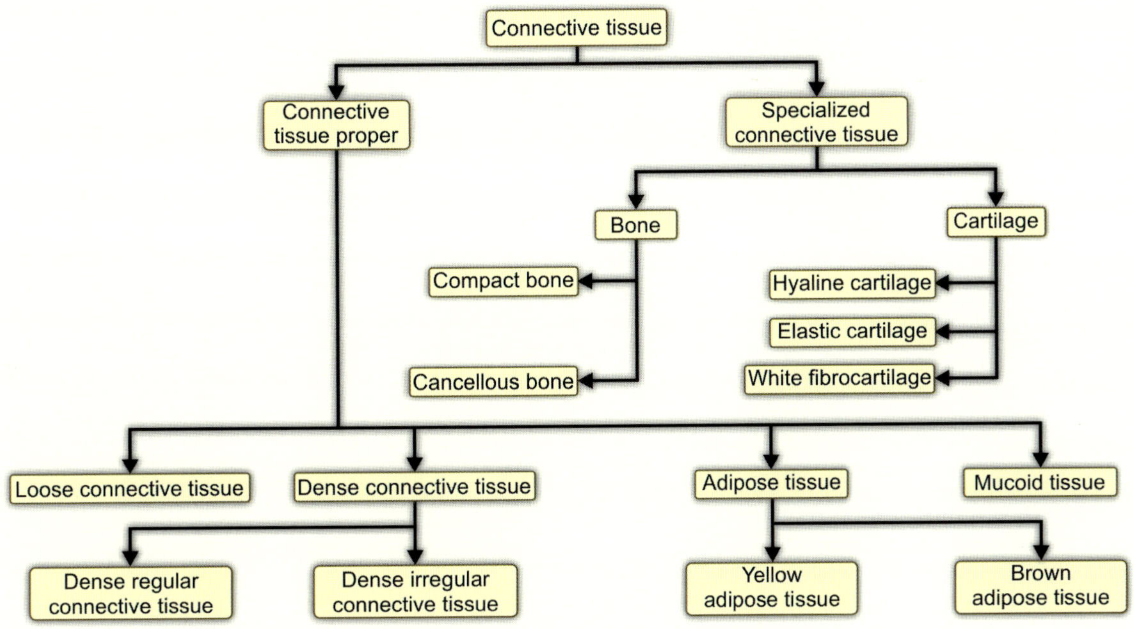

Figure 6.1: Classification of connective tissue

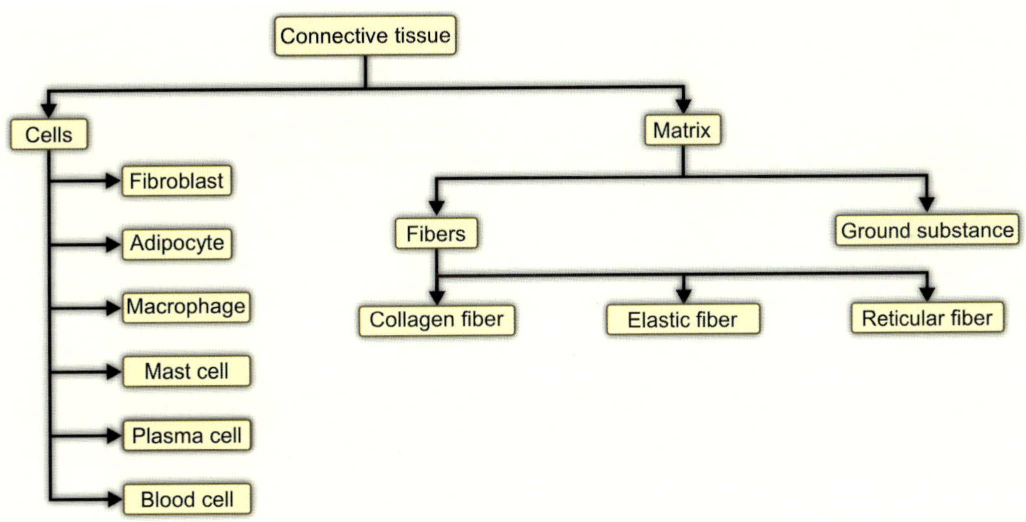

Figure 6.2: Constituents of connective tissue

- Adipose tissue is seen in two forms, i.e. yellow adipose tissue and brown adipose tissue.

Functions

- Acts as storehouse of nutrition.
- Acts as insulator.
- Acts as shock absorber.
- Gives cushing effect.

Macrophage (Fig. 6.5)

- This cell is also called **histocyte or clasmatocyte.**
- A macrophage is a large cell, which is oval to irregular shaped, with a kidney-shaped nucleus and large number of multiple granules in it.
- A macrophage is either a **motile cell** or **fixed cell**, i.e. motility of the cell depends upon the suitable stimulation. In some cases many macrophages fuse together, forming a multinucleated **giant cell.**

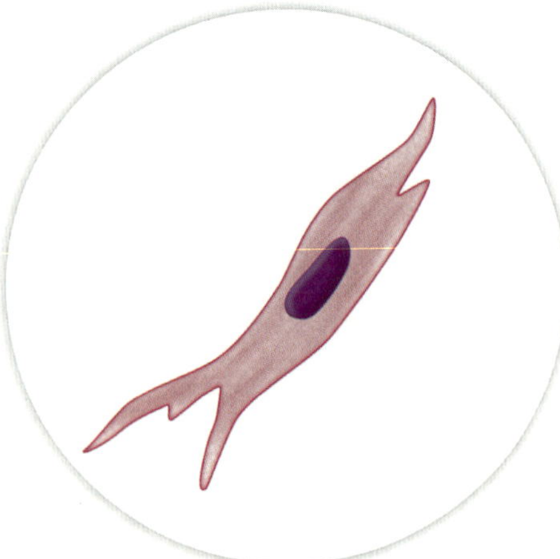

Figure 6.3: Fibroblast

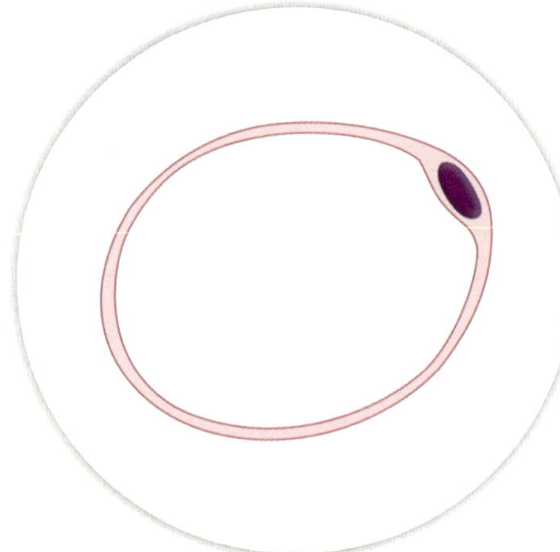

Figure 6.4: Adipocytes

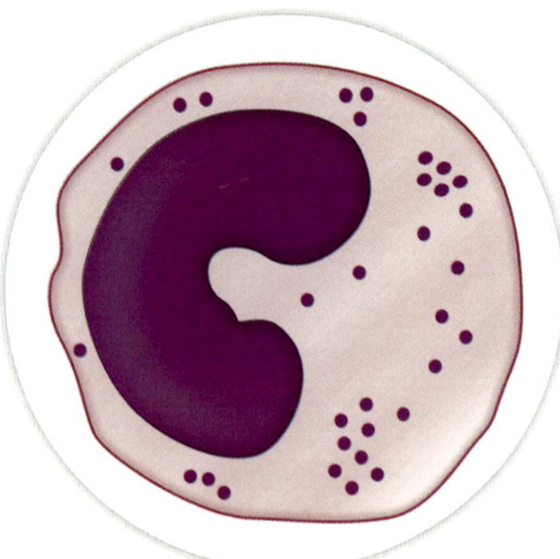

Figure 6.5: Macrophage

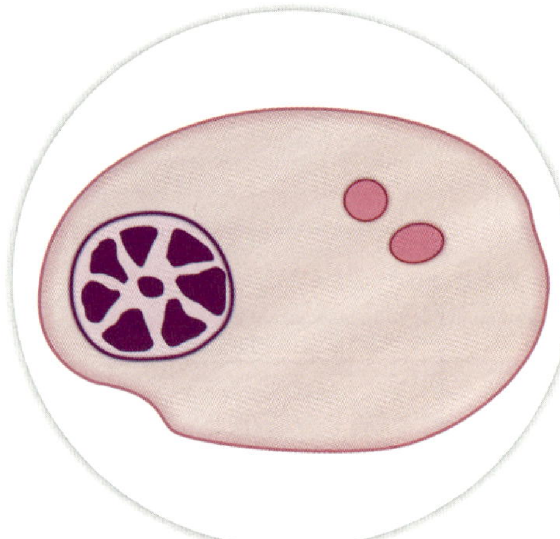

Figure 6.6: Plasma cell

- Macrophages are derived from the hemopoietic stem cells of the bone marrow and are included under **mononuclear phagocyte system**.
- A detailed picture of the cell structure can be demonstrated by **vital staining** technique.

Functions

- The most important function is to phagocytose the waste or foreign bodies, or particulate matter.
- They act like the **scavengers of the body**.
- They also take part in antigen-antibody reactions of the cell and thus play an important role in immunological mechanism.

Plasma Cell (Fig. 6.6)

- A plasma cell is a form of B-lymphocyte, which is a component of loose connective tissue as well as lymphoid tissue.
- Here the cell is small, rounded with eccentrically placed nucleus and the nucleus shows typical **cart wheel** appearance, because of its chromatin arrangement. The cytoplasm is highly basophilic due to the presence of rough endoplasmic reticulum.
- Here the cytoplasm of the cell contains many inclusion forms known as **Russell bodies** and are believed to be the stored form of antibodies of the cell.

Functions

- Plasma cells produce the immunoglobulin (antibodies).
- They play a great role in Modern Immunology.

Mast Cell (Fig. 6.7)

- A mast cell is a modified basophil, which is also called **mastocyte or histoaminocyte.**
- It is a round to oval-shaped cell with small, centrally placed nucleus.
- The cytoplasm of the cell is rich in metachromatic granules and are demonstrated by **periodic acid-Schiff (PAS) staining technique.**
- Based on staining principles they are believed to be acid mucopolysaccharides chemically.
- They are widely distributed in the connective tissue of the skin, along the blood vessels, digestive and respiratory organs.
- Mast cell produces **histamine and heparin.** It also produces various enzymes and other factors that attract the eosinophils and neutrophils.

Functions

- Histamine released by the mast cell takes part in allergic reaction and it also causes vasoconstriction of the blood vessels.
- Heparin is an another chemical substance released by the mast cell, which acts as an anticoagulant and helps in maintaining the fluidity of blood.
- Mast cells also take part in inflammation and healing mechanism of the body.

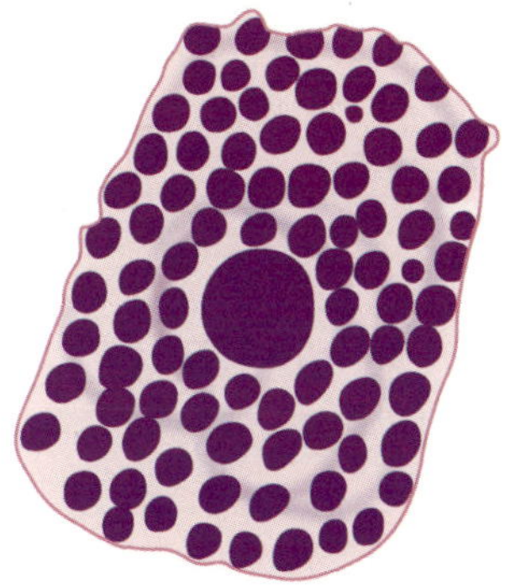

Figure 6.7: Mast cell

FIBERS OF THE CONNECTIVE TISSUE

Collagen Fiber (Figs 6.8A and B)

- They are also called **white fibers,** since they appear white in a fresh unstained preparation (Table 6.1).
- Collagen fibers are long, wavy bundles of fibers, which split into branches or anastomose with the adjacent bundles, but individual fibers will never branch.
- It is chemically made up of a protein called **collagen,** which in turn made up of repeated units of **tropocollagen.**
- When a beam of light is passed on collagen fibers, the light splits up into beams that are refracted in different directions and this phenomenon is known as **Birefringence phenomenon.**
- Collagen fiber is digested in the body by an enzyme **collaginase.**

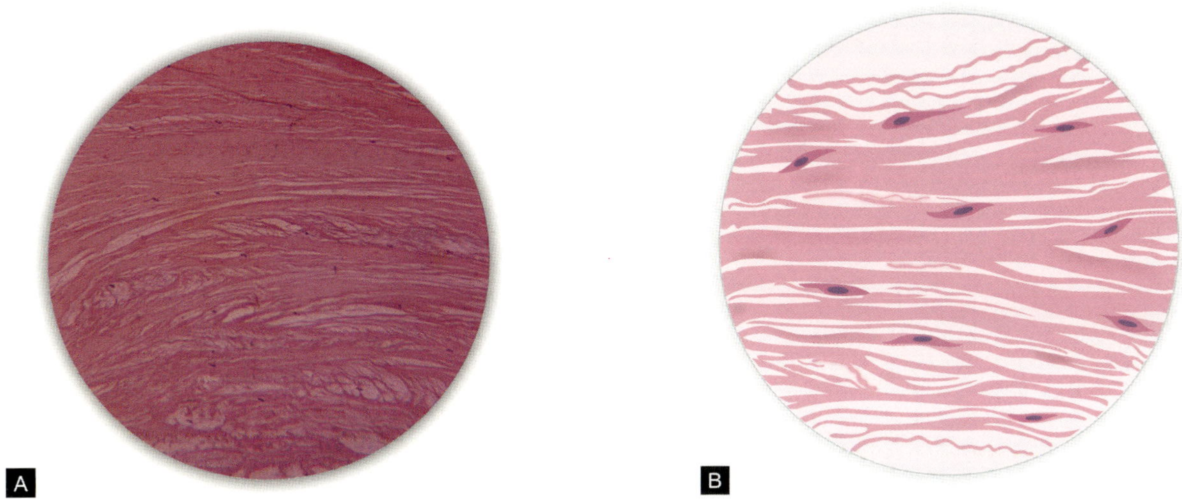

Figures 6.8A and B: Collagen fibers. **A.** Photograph; **B.** Diagrammatic representation.

Table 6.1: Staining characters of collagen fibers

Staining method	Stains
H and E	Light pink
Masson's trichome	Blue
Van Gieson	Pink
Silver impregnation	Brown

- There are more than 25 types of collagen fibers, which have been classified based on their molecular composition, morphological character, distribution and their function.

Types of Collagen Fiber

The important types are:

Type I: These are the collagen fibers of classical description having all the properties described above. They are found in connective tissue like bone, tendon, ligament, fasciae, aponeurosis and dermis of the skin.

Type II: Here, the collagen fibers are very minute and delicate in their structure and are mainly seen in hyaline cartilage.

Type III: Here, the collagen fibers are intermediate of both type I and type II fibers. This type of collagen fibers divides actively forming a network like structure, hence they are also referred as **reticular fibers**. They form the supporting network in many organs like spleen, lymph node, bone marrow, liver, kidney and most of the glands.

Elastic Fibers (Fig. 6.9)

- They are also called **yellow fibers** as they appear yellow in color in a fresh unstained preparation.
- Elastic fibers are short non-wavy, run singly, branch and anastomose with each other and they are thinner than collagen fibers.
- It is chemically made up of a protein called **elastin,** which in turn is made up of repeated units of **tropoelastin**.
- As the name itself indicates the elastic fibers are elastic in nature, can be stretched and return to their original length when tension is released. They do not show **Birefringence phenomenon**.
- Elastic fibers are digested in the body by an enzyme called **elastase.**
- Elastic fibers can be stained with **orcein, Weigert's resorcin fuchsin, Verhoeff's stain** and very faintly with **eosin**.

Occurrence

Ligamentum nuchae, ligamentum flavum, large arteries, loose areolar connective tissue and elastic cartilage, etc.

Reticular Fibers (Fig. 6.10)

- These fibers are nothing but the type III collagen fibers.
- Since they actively branch to form a delicate network, hence they are referred to as **reticular fiber** (refer type III collagen fibers for more details).

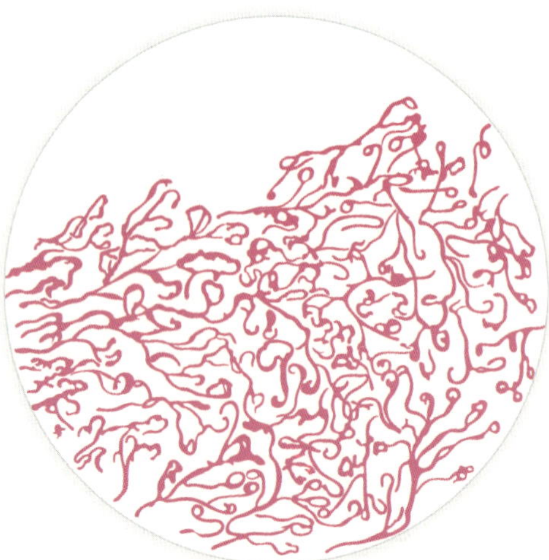

Figure 6.9: Elastic fibers

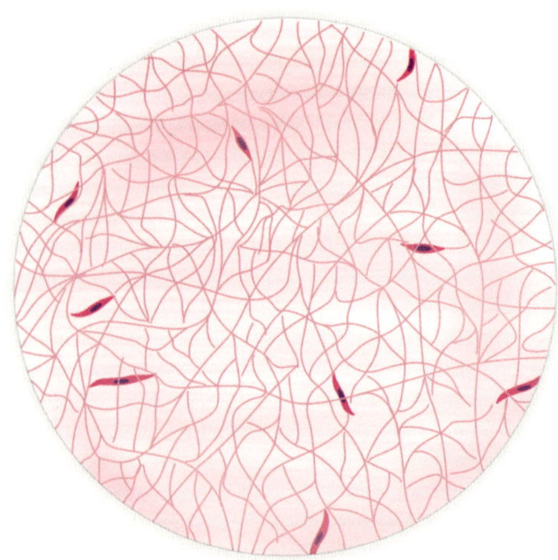

Figure 6.10: Reticular fibers

GROUND SUBSTANCE

- Ground substance is a clear amorphous, semisolid or jelly-like substance in which the cells are scattered.
- Presence of abundant ground substance is the characteristic feature of connective tissue.

Composition

- Ground substance is made up of 85%–90% of water and 10%–15% of solid particles.
- Solid particles include organic, inorganic and few gases. It is rich in mucopolysaccharides and their derivatives, which are responsible for the consistency and viscosity of the ground substance.
- The compositions of the ground substance are detailed in Figure 6.11.

Functions

- Nutritive in function.
- Supportive in function.
- Protective in function.

FUNCTIONS OF CONNECTIVE TISSUE

Different functions of the connective tissue are explained as follows:

- **Supportive:** Connective tissue gives structural and mechanical support to the body by connecting the cells, tissues and organs together.

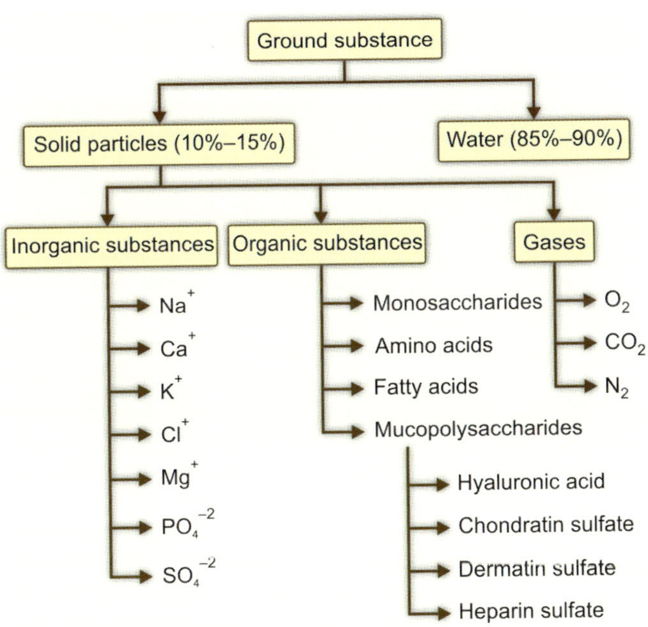

Figure 6.11: Compositions of ground substance

- **Transport:** Connective tissue matrix serves as a medium through which the nutrients and metabolites are exchanged between the cells and blood.
- **Packing:** The loose areolar connective tissue fills the gap in between the cells of various tissue and gives a proper shape to the organ.
- **Storage:** Adipocytes are rich in fat content, which acts as storehouse of energy. Loose areolar connective tissue also stores water and electrolytes.
- **Defense:** Most of the cells in connective tissue are involved in the defensive mechanism of the body either directly or indirectly.
- **Repair:** Connective tissue plays a major role in tissue healing and filling the gap in the wounds, injuries and infected areas.

DENSE CONNECTIVE TISSUE

Dense connective tissue is a type of connective tissue, which is rich in densely packed fibers with very few number of cells and ground substance.

Types

- **Dense irregular connective tissue:** It is rich in collagen fibers, which are arranged randomly in an irregular fashion along with few fibroblasts.
  Occurrence: Dermis of skin, capsule of different organs like spleen, liver, kidney, thymus, tunica adventitia of blood vessels and periosteum of the bone.
- **Dense regular connective tissue:** It is also rich in collagen fibers, which are arranged regularly with the parallel line along with few fibroblasts.
  Occurrence: Tendons and ligament.

LOOSE AREOLAR CONNECTIVE TISSUE

Slide No. 1

Identification Points

- Long wavy collagen fibers
- Short branching elastic fibers
- Different types of connective tissue cells.

Introduction

- This is a type of connective tissue, rich in cells with an abundant matrix. There is a loose and irregular arrangement of the connective tissue fibers in it, hence the name **loose connective tissue.**

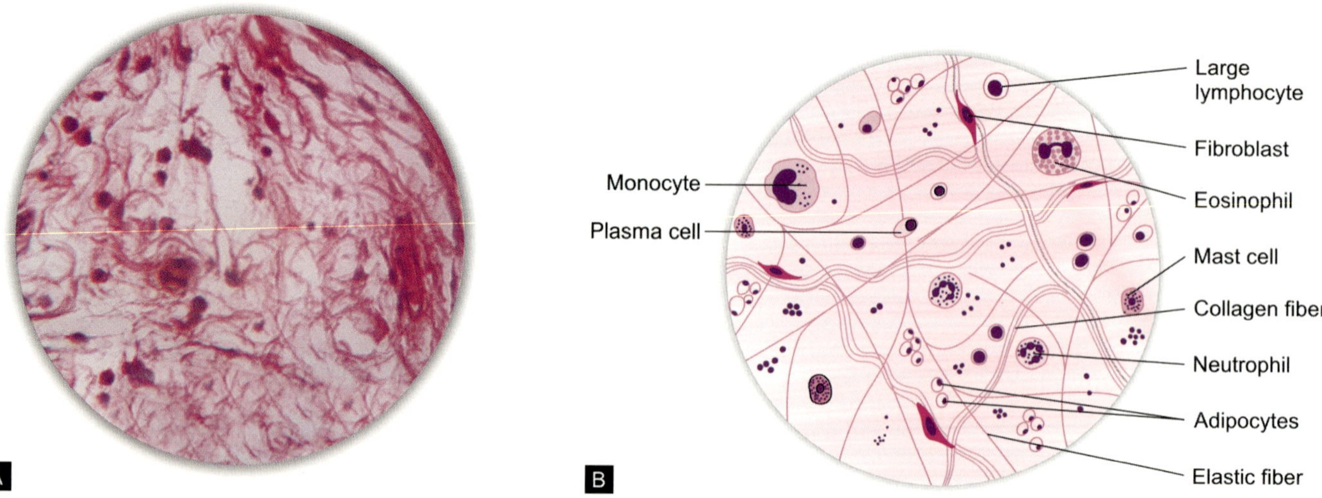

Figures 6.12A and B: Loose areolar connective tissue. **A.** Photograph; **B.** Diagrammatic representation.

- On examination few air spaces are also seen in the extracellular matrix, hence it is also called **loose areolar connective tissue** (Figs 6.12A and B).

Constituents of loose areolar connective tissue is same as that of a typical connective tissue (refer page No. 32).

Functions

- Helps in wound healing.
- Supportive in function.

Clinical Histology
Loose areolar connective tissue is seen in the scratched areas wounds of the skin and other organs, which later gives a brownish appearance over the surface
This fills up the gap in injured tissues, which later form the scar

Discussions

- What is loose areolar connective tissue?
- Name the cells present in loose connective tissue.
- Name the different fibers present in loose connective tissue.
- List the functions of fibroblast and mast cell.

ADIPOSE TISSUE

Slide No. 2

Identification Points

- Rounded/Oval/Polygonal cells
- Empty cells with scanty cytoplasm
- Peripherally situated nucleus.

Introduction

- Adipose tissue is a type of connective tissue, rich in adipocytes. Adipocytes are the fat cells, which are oval/rounded when occurring singly and polygonal in colonies (Figs 6.13A and B).
- There is a central fat with peripheral scanty cytoplasm and prominent eccentric nucleus.
- All the adipocytes are grouped together to form lobules and are supported by reticular fibers.
- Adipose tissue is derived from mesenchymal cells of yolk sac called **lipoblast.**
- In man, the fat present in adipocyte is in the form of **triglyceride** and it is rich in **oleic acid, linolic acid and palmitic acid.**
- During the preparation of slides, the fat content is washed away by the chemicals like xylene and benzene, hence the fat is not visible in the cells.
- Special stains like **sudan III, IV, black, oil red O and osmic acid** are used to stain the fat content in adipocytes.

Distribution

- Just below the skin in superficial fascia as **panniculus adiposus,** axilla, breast, buttocks, thigh, palm, foot, around the stomach, kidney, heart and intestine.
- However, it is absent in nipple, areola of breast, eyelids, scrotum and penis.

Types (Table 6.2)

- Brown adipose tissue.
- Yellow adipose tissue.

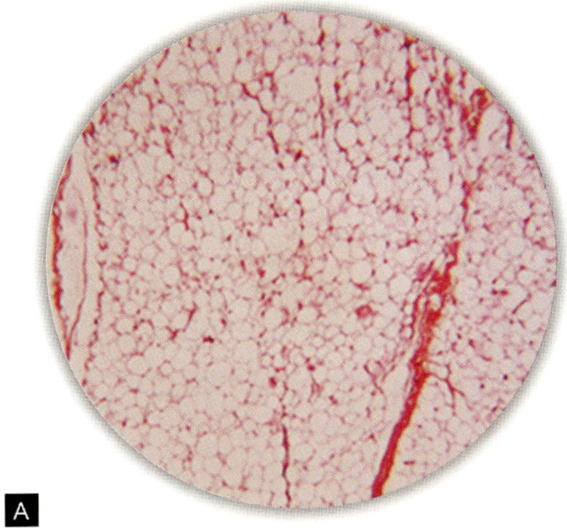

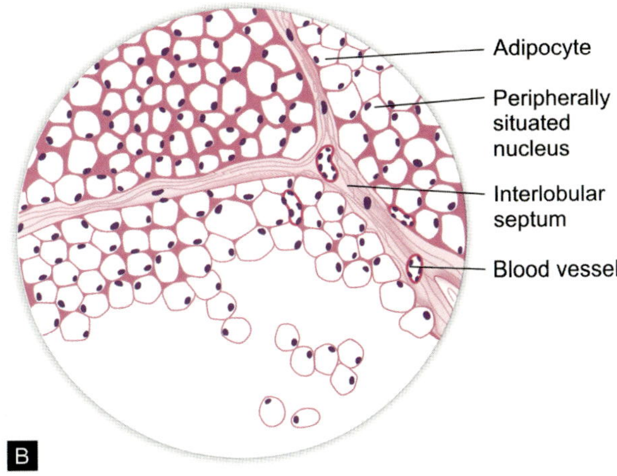

Figures 6.13A and B: Adipose tissue. **A.** Photograph; **B.** Diagrammatic representation.

Table 6.2: Difference between brown and yellow adipose tissues

Brown adipose tissue	Yellow adipose tissue
Found in children	Found in adults
Cells are smaller	Cells are larger
Cytoplasm and nucleus are not pushed to the periphery	Cytoplasm and nucleus are pushed to periphery
It is a multilocular adipose tissue	It is a unilocular adipose tissue
Contains numerous mitochondria	Contains less mitochondria
Associated with heat production	Associated with energy production

Functions

- Storehouse of nutrition.
- Acts as insulator.
- Acts as shock absorber.
- Gives cushing effect, etc.

Clinical Histology
Obesity in people is due to more and more accumulation of yellow adipose tissue in their body
Benign tumor of adipose tissue is called **lipoma**
Other forms of tumors are liposarcoma, lipochondroma, hibernoma, etc.

Discussions

- Why the adipocytes look empty?
- Why the nucleus of the cell is pushed to the periphery?
- Which germ layer gives rise to adipose tissue?
- What is the distribution of adipose tissue?
- Name some parts of the body where there is no adipose tissue.
- List the functions of adipose tissue.
- Name the special stains used to demonstrate the presence of fat in the adipose tissue.
- Differentiate between brown and yellow adipose tissue.
- What is blubber in whale?
- What is obesity?
- What is lipoma?

MUCOID TISSUE (Figs 6.14A and B)

Mucoid tissue is another type of (primititive) connective tissue with a jelly-like ground substance and an abundant amount of **hyaluronic acid**. It also contains peculiar star-shaped fibroblasts and delicate collagen fibers produced by it.

Occurrence: Umbilical cord, vitreous of eyeball.

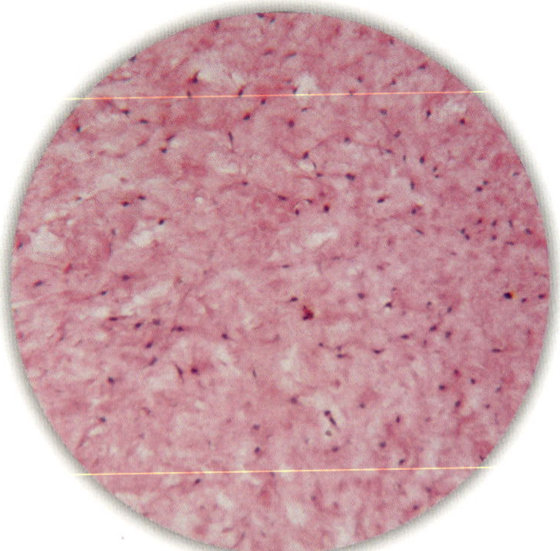

A

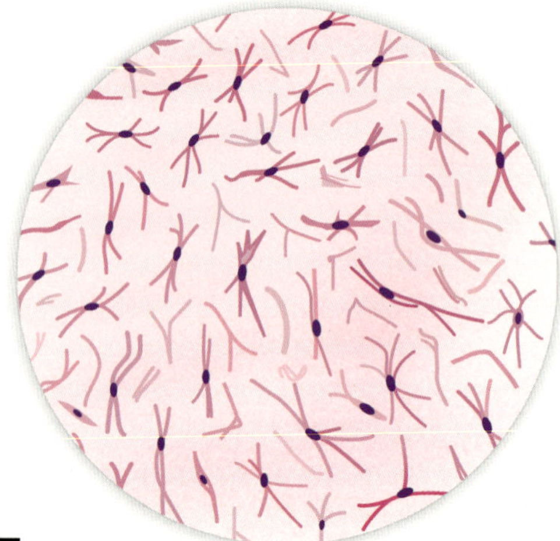

B

Figures 6.14A and B: Mucoid tissue. **A.** Photograph; **B.** Diagrammatic representation.

CHAPTER

7

Specialized Connective Tissue

BONE AND CARTILAGE

Even though, skeletal tissue is a part of connective tissue, but still it differs in its structure, function and mode of development; therefore, it is considered as specialized connective tissue.

The skeletal tissue is of two types (Fig. 7.1):

- Bone.
- Cartilage.

Bone

- Bone is a hard, but hollow connective tissue.
- It forms the skeletal framework in mammals.
- It is **mesodermal** in origin; most of the bones develop from the cartilage by **endochondral ossification**. But few bones develop directly from fibrous membrane by **intramembranous ossification**. Histologically, bone is classified into two types, i.e. compact bone and cancellous bone.

Cartilage

- Cartilage is a hard, but flexible connective tissue, which is also called **gristle**.

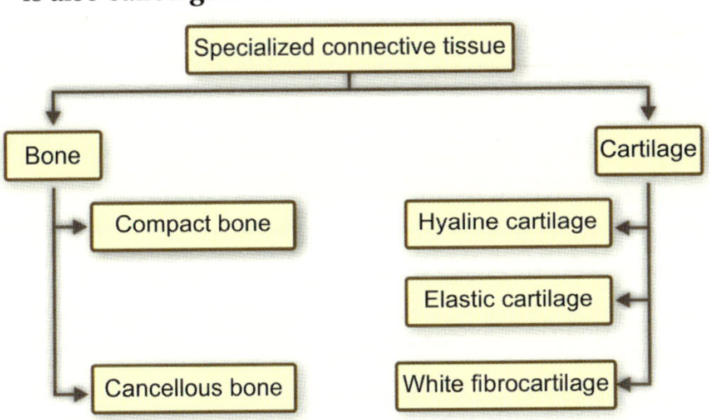

Figure 7.1: Classification of specialized connective tissue

- Cartilage forms the skeletal framework in the developing embryo and also seen in some parts of the body.
- Embryologically, cartilage is also derived from the **mesenchyme**.
- Unlike bone, cartilage is devoid of direct blood supply (except fibrocartilage).

There are three types of cartilage:

- Hyaline cartilage.
- Elastic cartilage.
- White fibrocartilage.

COMPACT BONE (TS) (Figs 7.2A and B)

Slide No. 3

Identification Points

- Presence of haversian system
- Haversian canal containing blood vessels
- Different types of lamellae.

COMPACT BONE (LS) (Figs 7.3A and B)

Slide No. 4

Identification Points

- Longitudinal sections of haversian canals
- Horizontal sections of Volkmann's canal
- Lamellae parallel to haversian canal.

COMPACT BONE (TS AND LS)

Introduction

- Compact bone is a hard tissue, usually seen in the shaft of the long bones surrounding the medullary cavity.

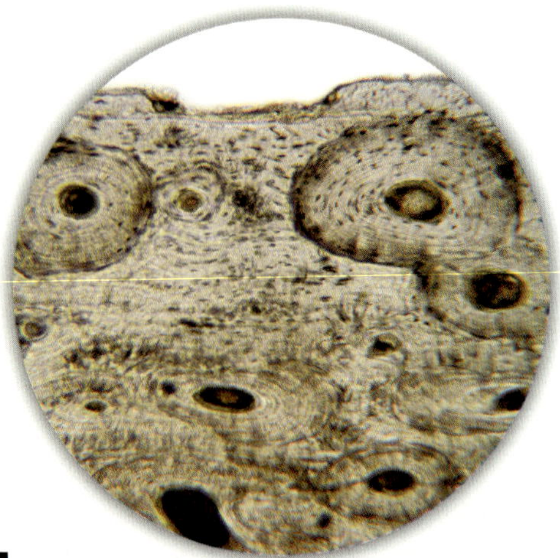

A

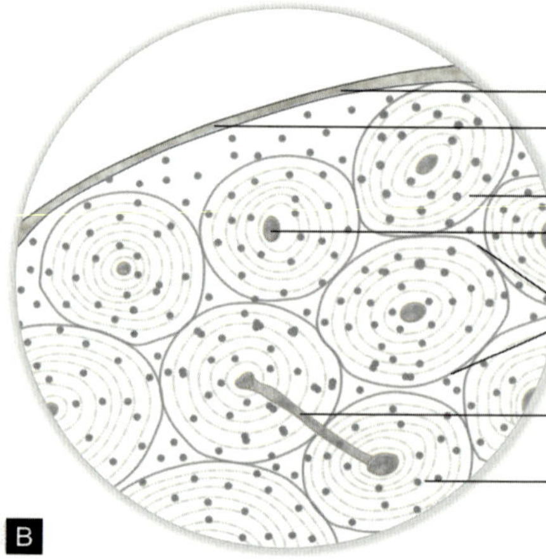

B

Figures 7.2A and B: Compact bone [transverse section (TS)]. **A.** Photograph; **B.** Diagrammatic representation.

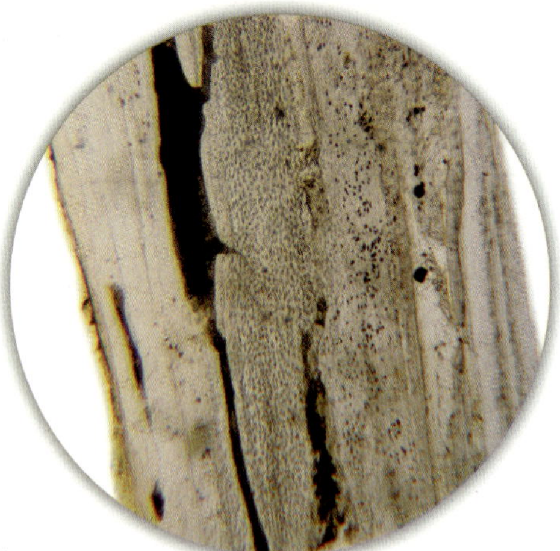

A

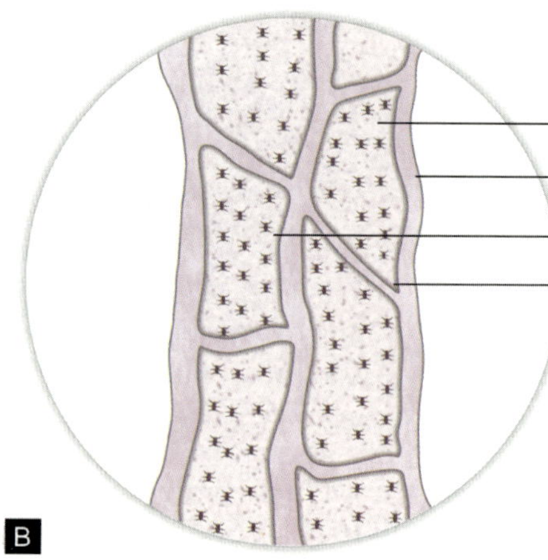

B

Figures 7.3A and B: Compact bone [longitudinal section (LS)]. **A.** Photograph; **B.** Diagrammatic representation.

- The presence of **Haversian system** is the characteristic feature of mammalian compact bone.

Structure

Transverse section of a compact bone shows the following features.

Extracellular Matrix

- Extracellur matrix consists of an amorphous homogeneous ground substance and fibers embedded in it.
- Ground substance consists of water and glycosaminoglycans and with special glycoproteins **osteonectin** and **osteocalcin**.
- It is also rich in calcium phosphate and calcium oxalate in the form of hydroxyapatite; hence the ground substance of compact bone is very hard and different than the usual ones.
- Ground substance is rich in type I collagen fibers, which gives lamellar appearance. Here, the collagen fiber is synthesized by the osteoblast cells.

Haversian System

Haversian system is the structural and functional unit of the mammalian compact bone. It is also called **osteon**. It can be explained under the following headings.

Haversian canal

- At the center of each haversian system, there is a canal called **haversian canal** (Fig. 7.4).
- It contains blood vessels and nerve fibers in it.

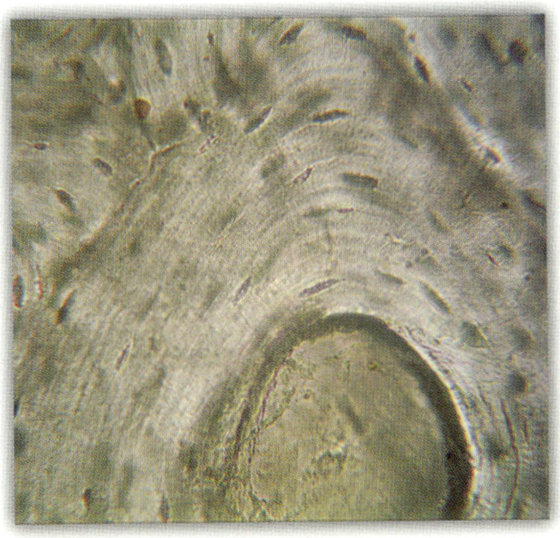

Figure 7.4: Haversian canal

Lamellae

- There are many concentric ring-like structures around the haversian canal called **lamellae**.
- It is made up of thin layer of collagen fibers and part of the ground substance.
- In between the two lamellae, there are many lacunae containing bone cells.

Types of lamellae

- **Concentric lamellae:** These are the typical lamellae seen in the haversian system. On an average of 2–20 lamellae are seen in a haversian system.
- **Interstitial lamellae:** These are seen in between the haversian system and they are the remnants of older haversian system, which were eroded during the bone remodeling, hence haversian canals are not seen in such lamellae.
- **Circumferential lamellae:** These are arranged in parallel bundles, which surround the whole bone. If they are found deep to the periosteum, they are referred as **outer circumferential lamellae**. If found near the endosteum, they are referred as **inner circumferential lamellae**.

Lacuna

- Lacuna is a space or sac-like structure, which encloses the bone cell in it.
- Each bone cell is connected to an another bone cell by the extension of the cytoplasmic threads which passes through the minute canals of matrix known as **canaliculi** (Fig. 7.5). They help in exchanging and transportation of nutrition and waste matters from cell to cell.

Bone cells

A typical bone cell is a star-shaped structure enclosed within the lacuna.

Types of bone cell:

- **Osteoprogenitor cells:** These are the basic stem cells derived from the mesenchyme of the yolk sac, which converts themselves into osteoblasts. They are seen over inner and outer bone surfaces.
- **Osteoblasts:** These are cuboidal shaped immature bone cells capable of producing collagen fibers and the extracellular matrix. They are usually seen wherever there is bone formation.
- **Osteocytes:** These are star-shaped mature bone cells formed from osteoblasts. They are seen in haversian system and interstitial lamellae; their exact function is not known, but it is believed that their function is to maintain the bone tissue.
- **Osteoclasts:** These are the large irregular multinucleated giant cells, which mainly take part in the resorption of the bone. They are found at the site of bone resorption called **resorption bays** or **Howship's lacunae**.

Cement line

Cement line is a refractile of modified bone matrix with a basophilic zone, which forms a boundary between the two adjacent osteons.

Volkmann's Canal

- Longitudinal section of a compact bone show many horizontal connections between the haversian canals of osteons and are referred as **Volkmann's canal** (Fig. 7.6).
- They contain the blood vessels and nerve fibers in it.

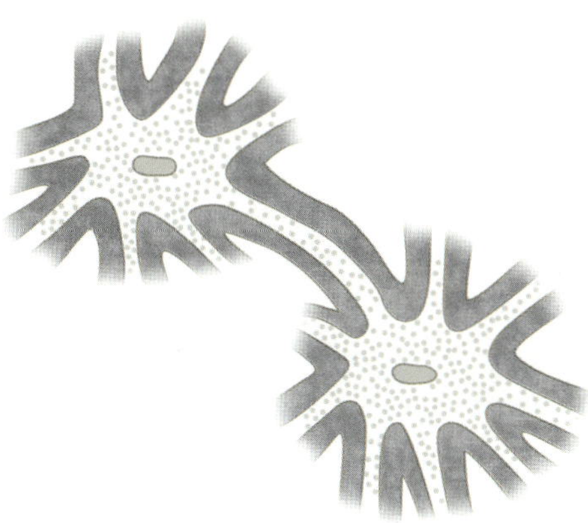

Figure 7.5: Canaliculi

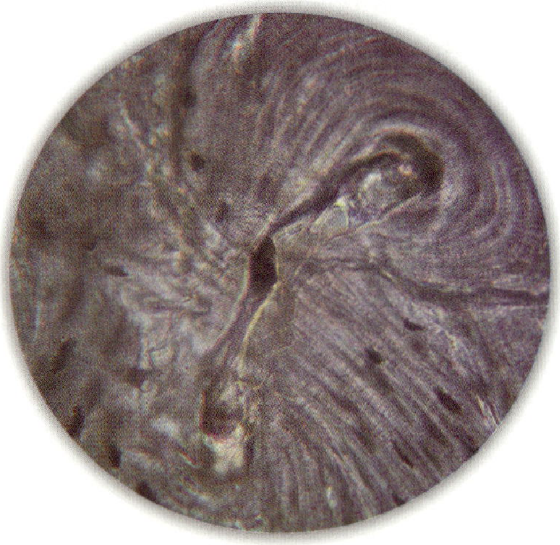

Figure 7.6 : Volkmann's canal

Functions of Bone

- Forms skeletal framework in mammals
- Acts as storehouse of calcium
- Helps in locomotion
- Forms the site of erythropoiesis
- Acts as one of the important reticuloendothelial systems in body
- Bone is a primary lymphoid organ and produces T lymphocytes.

Discussions

- Why is the cellular matrix of bone different than the usual ones?
- Which cells secrete the extracellular matrix and fibers in the bone?
- What is haversian systems? What is its another name?
- What are lamellae? Name its different types.
- Name the different types of bone cells, location and their functions.
- What are canaliculi?
- What is cement line?
- What is lacuna and what does it contain?
- What are the differences between Volkmann's canal and haversian canal?
- List the functions of bone.

HYALINE CARTILAGE (Gr 'Hyalos'—glass)

Slide No. 5

Identification Points

- Outermost perichondrium
- Homogeneous matrix
- Chondrocytes forming cell nests.

Introduction

- As the name itself indicates, the cartilage is characterized by the presence of an amorphous, homogeneous protoplasm resembling the glass. Hence, hyaline cartilage (Figs 7.7A and B) is also called **glass cartilage**.
- In general, any cartilage is derived from the mesenchyme of the yolk sac forming different types of cartilages.

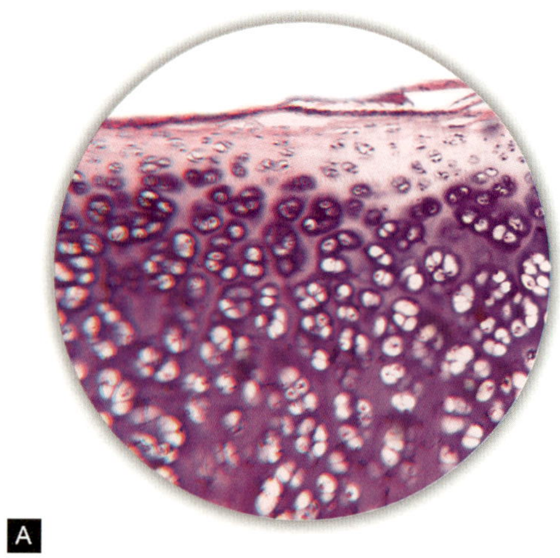

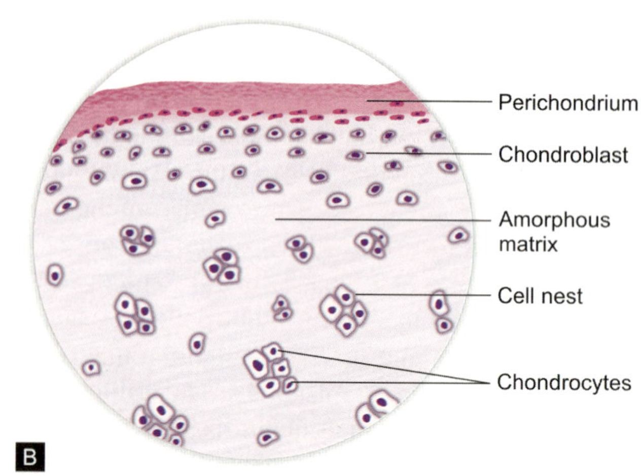

Figures 7.7A and B: Hyaline cartilage. **A.** Photograph; **B.** Diagrammatic representation.

Structure

A typical structure of hyaline cartilage is explained as follows.

Matrix

The matrix consists of two parts, i.e. ground substance and fibers.

Ground substance

- Ground substance is an amorphous semi-solid, gel-like material rich in glycosaminoglycans with abundant amount of chondroitin sulfate in it.
- Ground substance of hyaline cartilage is highly basophilic and periodic acid-Schiff (PAS)-positive in nature.

Fibers

- Matrix of hyaline cartilage is rich in type II collagen fibers, which are produced by chondroblasts.
- Even though matrix is rich in collagen fibers, but still it appears homogeneous. It is because the refractive index of type II collagen fiber is same as that of the ground substance.

Different forms of matrix

- Territorial matrix: This is newly formed matrix seen immediately surrounding the cartilage cells and does not contain any fibers in it. Thus, it appears more basophilic.
- Interterritorial matrix: It is an old matrix seen in the spaces or areas between the cell nests and is rich in fibers; hence, it appears less basophilic.

Perichondrium

- Perichondrium is a special form of dense irregular connective tissue found in covering the free surface of the hyaline cartilage.
- It is rich in fibers, fibroblasts and blood vessels.
- Since the hyaline cartilage is avascular in nature; hence, it gets its nutrition from the perichondrium by simple diffusion.

Cellular Part

Following type of cells are seen in the hyaline cartilage:

- **Chondrogenic cells:** These are undifferentiated, flat cells seen in the inner layer of perichondrium. They have the capacity of proliferating and differentiating into chondroblasts.
- **Chondroblasts:** These are the immature cartilaginous cells seen very close to the perichondrium. They are short, small, elongated cells, rich in all the cell organelle in it and usually occur singly or individually:
  - Chondroblasts are covered by a sac-like structure called **lacunae**.
  - They produce the extracellular matrix including the type II collagen fibers.
- **Chondrocytes:** These are the matured form of cartilaginous cells seen away from the perichondrium:
  - A chondrocyte is a large oval-shaped cell with relatively less cell organelle in it. Usually the cells are seen in a group forming **cell nests or isogenous cell groups**.
  - They undergo ossification process finally converting themselves into bone cells.

Occurrence

Hyaline cartilage is seen in costal cartilage, articular surface of most of the synovial joints, thyroid cartilage, cricoids cartilage and arytenoid cartilage of the larynx, skeletal framework of the fetus, tracheal rings, epiphyseal plate of the bone, articular surface of the sesamoid bone, parts of the nasal septum and lateral wall of the nose, etc.

Functions

- Hyaline cartilage mainly forms skeleton of the developing embryo.
- It also gives a proper shape to the nose and other parts.
- Prevents the friction between the two articular surfaces of the bones.
- Responsible for the formation of bone by endochondral ossification, etc.

Discussions

- Why hyaline cartilage is also called glass cartilage?
- Matrix of hyaline cartilage appears homogeneous amorphous. Give reason.
- What is perichondrium? What is its function?
- Name the different types of cells seen in the hyaline cartilage.
- Which cell is responsible for the production of matrix including the fibers?
- What is cell nest or isogenous cell group?
- What is the difference between lacuna of the bone and lacuna of the cartilage?
- List the occurrence of hyaline cartilage in the body.
- Describe the functions of hyaline cartilage.
- What is endochondral ossification?

ELASTIC CARTILAGE

Slide No. 6

Identification Points

- Outer perichondrium
- Matrix rich in elastic fibers
- Numerous chondrocytes in matrix.

Introduction

- Elastic cartilage (Figs 7.8A and B) is a type of cartilage, which is almost similar to that of hyaline cartilage with respect to the perichondrium, cellular pattern, matrix composition and its development.
- The only main difference is matrix of elastic cartilage is rich in elastic fibers, hence the name given **elastic cartilage**.

Structure

Extracellular matrix

- Since the extracellular matrix of elastic cartilage is rich in elastic fibers, which are dispersed randomly, hence the matrix of the elastic cartilage is not homogeneous like hyaline cartilage.
- Composition of the matrix in elastic cartilage is almost same as that of hyaline cartilage.
- There is an outermost perichondrium seen in elastic cartilage, which is nutritive in nature. Even the cellular pattern is same as that of hyaline cartilage provided, elastic cartilage is rich with numerous chondrocytes.

Occurrence

Elastic cartilage is seen in external ear pinna, epiglottis, external auditory meatus, auditory tube, corniculate and cuneiform cartilage, etc.

Discussions

- Which fiber is rich in the matrix of elastic cartilage?
- List the differences between hyaline cartilage and elastic cartilage.
- Name the occurrence of elastic cartilage.

FIBROCARTILAGE

Slide No. 7

Identification Points

- Absence of perichondrium
- Matrix rich in collagen fibers
- Minimal cells arranged in rows.

Introduction

- On naked examination, this type of cartilage looks like a dense fibrous tissue. Hence, it is called **fibrocartilage** (Figs 7.9A and B).
- Fibrocartilage is characterized by the presence of dense collagen or white fibers. Hence, it is also known as **white fibrocartilage**.

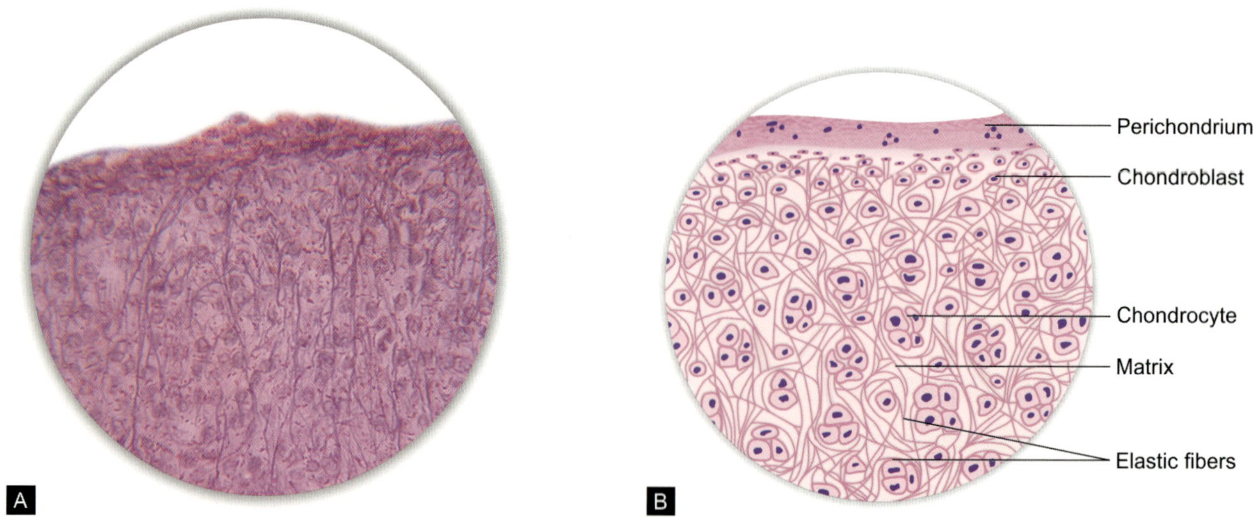

Figures 7.8A and B: Elastic cartilage. **A.** Photograph; **B.** Diagrammatic representation.

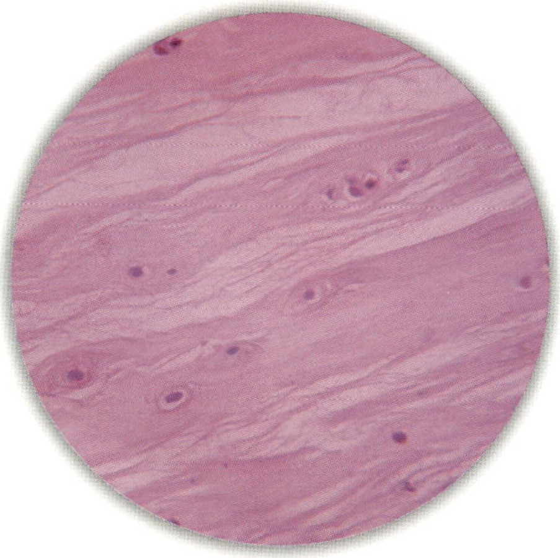

A

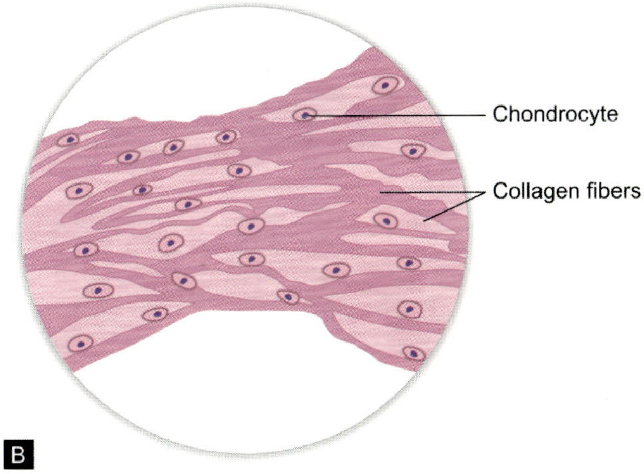

B

Figures 7.9A and B: Fibrocartilage. **A.** Photograph; **B.** Diagrammatic representation.

Structure

Extracellular matrix

- It is very scanty in fibrocartilage, since whole of the cartilage is filled by long wavy bundles of type I collagen fiber; hence, white fibers or collagen fibers occupy the whole of the matrix.
- Absence of perichondrium is the characteristic feature of white fibrocartilage. Therefore, it gets its nutrition directly from the blood vessels supplying it.
- Chondrocytes are very few and usually occur single or in a row here and there.

Occurrence

Intervertebral disks, menisci and articular disks, glenoid labrum, acetabular labrum, pubic symphyses and manubriosternal joint.

Discussions

- Which type of collagen fibers are rich in white fibrocartilage?
- Where do you see white fibrocartilage?

CHAPTER 8

Muscular Tissue

INTRODUCTION

- Muscular tissue is an important tissue in the body, which made the man to be the most powerful and strongest living entity on the earth.
- It also plays major role in locomotion of the body.

GENERAL FEATURES OF MUSCULAR TISSUE

- Muscular tissue is made up of repeated units of cell called **myocyte**.
- A myocyte is either long cylindrical or spindle-shaped structure, which usually appears like a fiber. Hence, most commonly it is referred as **muscle fiber.**
- The cell membrane surrounding the muscle fiber is known as **sarcolemma,** whereas **sarcoplasm** is the term given to its cytoplasm.
- The mitochondria and smooth endoplasmic reticulum of the muscle cell are named as **sarcosomes** and **sarcoplasmic reticulum** respectively.
- Each muscle fiber contains numerous thread like structures in it called **Myofibrils,** which is made up of different types of muscle proteins.
- **Actin, myosin, troponin, tropomycin actinin, titin, desmin, myogen** and **myoglobin** are the muscle proteins out of which actin, myosin, troponin and tropomycins take part in contraction and relaxation of muscle fibers hence they are referred to as **contractile proteins.**

CLASSIFICATION OF MUSCULAR TISSUE

Muscular tissue is classified as major and minor muscular tissue (Fig. 8.1).

Major muscular tissues are:

- Skeletal muscle.
- Visceral muscle.
- Cardiac muscle.

Minor muscular tissue includes:

- Myoepitheliocytes.
- Myofibroblasts.

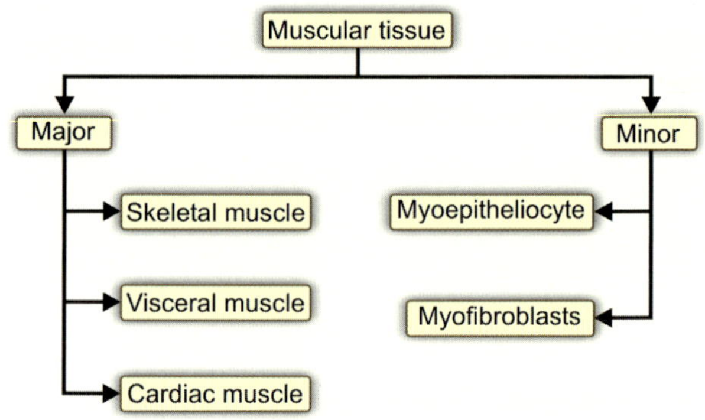

Figure 8.1: Classification of muscular tissue

SKELETAL MUSCLE (LS) (Figs 8.2A and B)

Slide No. 8

Identification Points

- Long cylindrical muscle cells
- Alternative dark and light bands
- Multinuclei at the periphery.

Introduction

- Skeletal muscles are the group of muscles, which form 40% to 50% of the body weight.
- Since they are always in association with skeletal system, hence named as **skeletal muscle.**
- Action of the skeletal muscle is under one's will and wish, so, they are also called **voluntary muscles.**

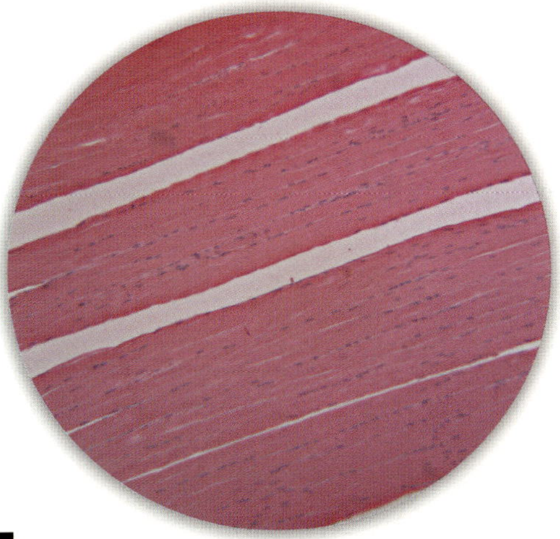

A

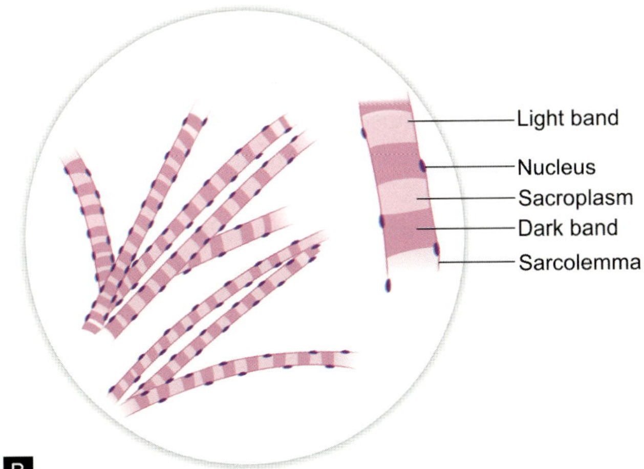

B

Figures 8.2A and B: Skeletal muscle [longitudinal section (LS)]. **A.** Photograph; **B.** Diagrammatic representation.

- These muscles have numerous striations or strips on its surface. Hence, it is also being referred as striped or **striated muscle.**

Longitudinal section (LS) of skeletal muscle can be explained under the following headings.

Muscle fiber

- It is a long cylindrical fiber like structure, which runs in parallel with other muscle fibers forming a **bundle** or **fasciculi.**
- In between the muscle fibers there is a thin layer of connective tissue with minute blood vessels and nerves running along their course.
- A skeletal muscle fiber is highly variable in its measurements. Length of it may vary from few millimeter to 35 cm as in case of sartorius muscle and width from 10 to 100 mm.
- Alternate dark and light bands are seen on the surface of skeletal muscle fiber, which is the most striking feature of it.
- Nucleus of the muscle fiber is long flat, which is seen peripherally just beneath the sarcolemma.
- Whereas sarcoplasm of the cell contains numerous minute thread-like structures called myofibrils.

Myofibril

- Myofibril is a part of muscle fiber seen in the sarcoplasm of the muscle cell.
- A typical myofibril is also long elongated cylindrical structure with alternate dark and light bands on it. Here the dark band is known as **A band** and light band is known as **I band.**
- A band has a narrow lighter area at its middle, which forms **H-zone.**
- M-line is seen in the middle of the H-zone, which indicates the middle part of myosin filament.
- Similarly, I band is also equally divided by a line called Z-line and this represents the middle part of the actin filament.

Sarcomere: It is the area found between two **Z-line** of the myofibril and it is **the structural and functional unit of the muscle fiber:**

- Ultrastructure of muscle fiber shows that the whole sarcolemma is filled with myofibrils, which pushes the nucleus of the cell toward periphery.
- In between the two myofibrils there exists **sarcoplasmic reticulum** with **sarcosomes** and few **glycogen stored granules.**

Functions

- Skeletal muscles help in locomotion of the body.
- It is the second storehouse of glycogen next to liver.
- It also acts as store of calcium.

Discussions

- What are the different names of skeletal muscle and give reason?
- What is the measurement of a typical skeletal muscle?
- What is the characteristic feature of skeletal muscle?
- Why the nucleus of cell is pushed to periphery?

- Explain the terms sarcolemma, sarcoplasm, sarcoplasmic reticulum and sarcosomes.
- What is a myofibril?
- Name the muscle proteins. Which muscle proteins are called contractile muscle proteins?
- Why is the alternate dark and light band due to?
- What is sarcomere?
- List the functions of skeletal muscles.

Clinical Histology
Reduction in the number and size of muscle cell is called **muscular atrophy** and is seen in old age people.
Increase in the size of a muscle cell without increase in its number is called **muscular hypertrophy.**
Increase in the number of muscle cell leads to muscular hyperplasia. Physiologically, **muscular hypertrophy** and hyperplasia is seen in pregnant women.
Myasthenia gravis is an autoimmune disorder where autoantibodies are developed against muscular end plate resulting in its destruction and muscular weakness.

SKELETAL MUSCLE (TS) (Figs 8.3A and B)

Slide No. 9

Identification Points

- Peripherally nucleated muscle fibers in bundles or fascicles
- Perimysium around the muscle fascicles
- Epimysium covering the whole muscle tissue.

  A cross section of the skeletal muscle shows:
- Numerous muscle fibers covered by a protective membrane called **endomysium.**
- Many muscle fibers unit to form bundles or fasciculi, which is surrounded by a connective tissue forming **perimysium.**
- Many muscular bundles or fasciculi unite to form a muscular tissue (muscle), which, in turn, is enclosed by a dense connective tissue rich in reticular fibers and is called **epimysium.**

Types of Muscle Fibers

There are two types of skeletal muscle fibers called red and white muscle fibers and it can be explained (Table 8.1).

Table 8.1: Types of skeletal muscle fibers

Red muscle fiber	White muscle fiber
Rich in myoglobin and cytochrome	Contains less myoglobin and cytochrome
Numerous mitochondria are present in it	Only few mitochondria are present in it
Not easily fatigued on repeated contractions	Easily fatigued on repeated contractions
Has good blood supply, e.g. postural muscles	Has poor blood supply, e.g. extraocular muscles

Discussions

- What is an endomysium?
- What is an epimysium?
- What is a perimysium?
- Name the different types of skeletal muscle fibers.
- List the differences between red muscle fibers and white muscle fibers.

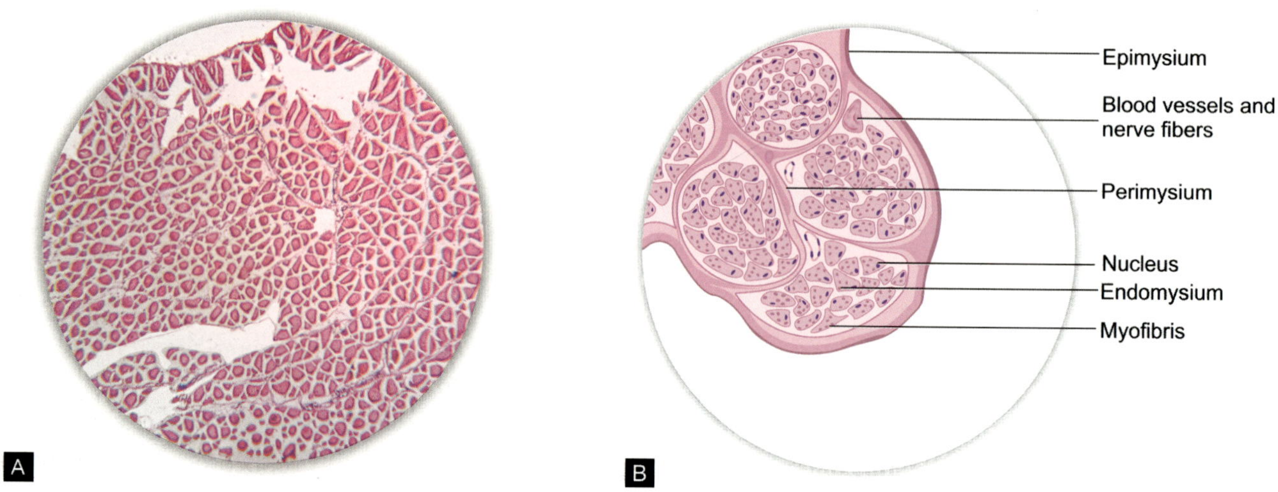

Figures 8.3A and B: Skeletal muscle [transverse section (TS)]. **A.** Photograph; **B.** Diagrammatic representation.

SMOOTH MUSCLE (LS) (Fig. 8.4)

Slide No. 10

Identification Points

- Long spindle-shaped myocytes in bundle
- Absence of striations
- Centrally flat oval nucleus.

Introduction

- Smooth muscle fibers are the long elongated spindle-shaped structures seen in musculature of blood vessels and visceral organs. Hence, called **visceral muscles.**
- Since the action of the smooth muscle cell is not under one's will and wish hence, another name **involuntary muscle.**

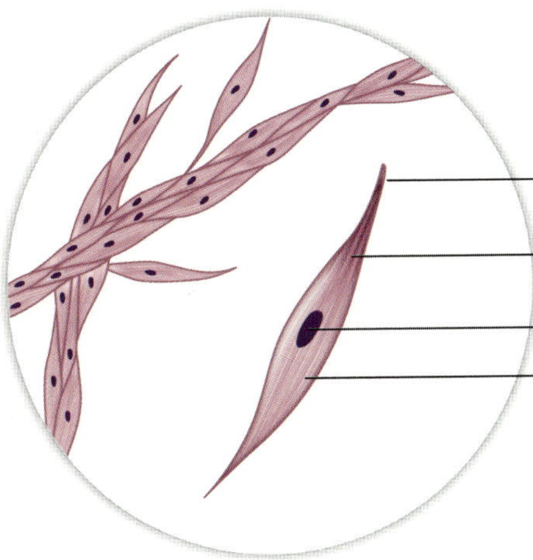

Figure 8.4: Smooth muscles (LS) (Diagrammatic representation)

- Smooth muscles are characterized by the absence of bands or striation hence, it is also being referred as **non-striated muscle.**
- As mentioned above a smooth muscle cell is a spindle-shaped cell with a pointed end on either side, usually measuring from 30 to 500 mm in length.
- Each smooth muscle cell is made up of a centrally placed oval nucleus, seen in the cytoplasm (sarcoplasm) and is covered by a plasma membrane (sarcolemma).
- The sarcoplasm of the cell contains numerous thread-like structures in it and are named as myofibrils.
- Here each myocyte is connected to another myocyte by a gap junction thus forming many muscular bundles or fasciculi.

Functions

- Smooth muscles present in blood vessels contract and help in blood circulation.
- Smooth muscles of the gut system initiate peristalsis thus helping in fast absorption of food, etc.

Discussions

- What are the other names for smooth muscle? Why are they called so?
- Describe a smooth muscle cell.
- List the functions of smooth muscle in the body.

CARDIAC MUSCLE (LS) (Figs 8.5A to D)

Slide No. 11

Identification Points

- Short cylindrical muscle fibers
- Centrally placed nucleus
- Presence of intercalated disks.

Introduction

Cardiac muscle is a special type of muscle, which is seen exclusively in myocardium of the heart. Though its morphological features resemble that of skeletal muscles, it functions like involuntary muscles.

Structure

- A typical cardiac muscle is a short cylindrical muscle fiber with a branching pattern.
- It also bears alternate dark and light bands, but they are not clearly visible under light microscope.
- Each muscle cell has a central oval nucleus with an abundant mitochondria in it and it is also supplied by numerous blood vessels.
- Presence of **intercalated disk** is the special feature of cardiac muscle, which helps in transmission of nerve impulses from one muscle to another thus contracting simultaneously. Hence, cardiac muscle is said to be a **functional syncytium.**
- It also obeys **all or none law.**

Functions

Cardiac muscle present in the heart contracts continuously in a regular fashion thus keeps the blood in circulation throughout the body.

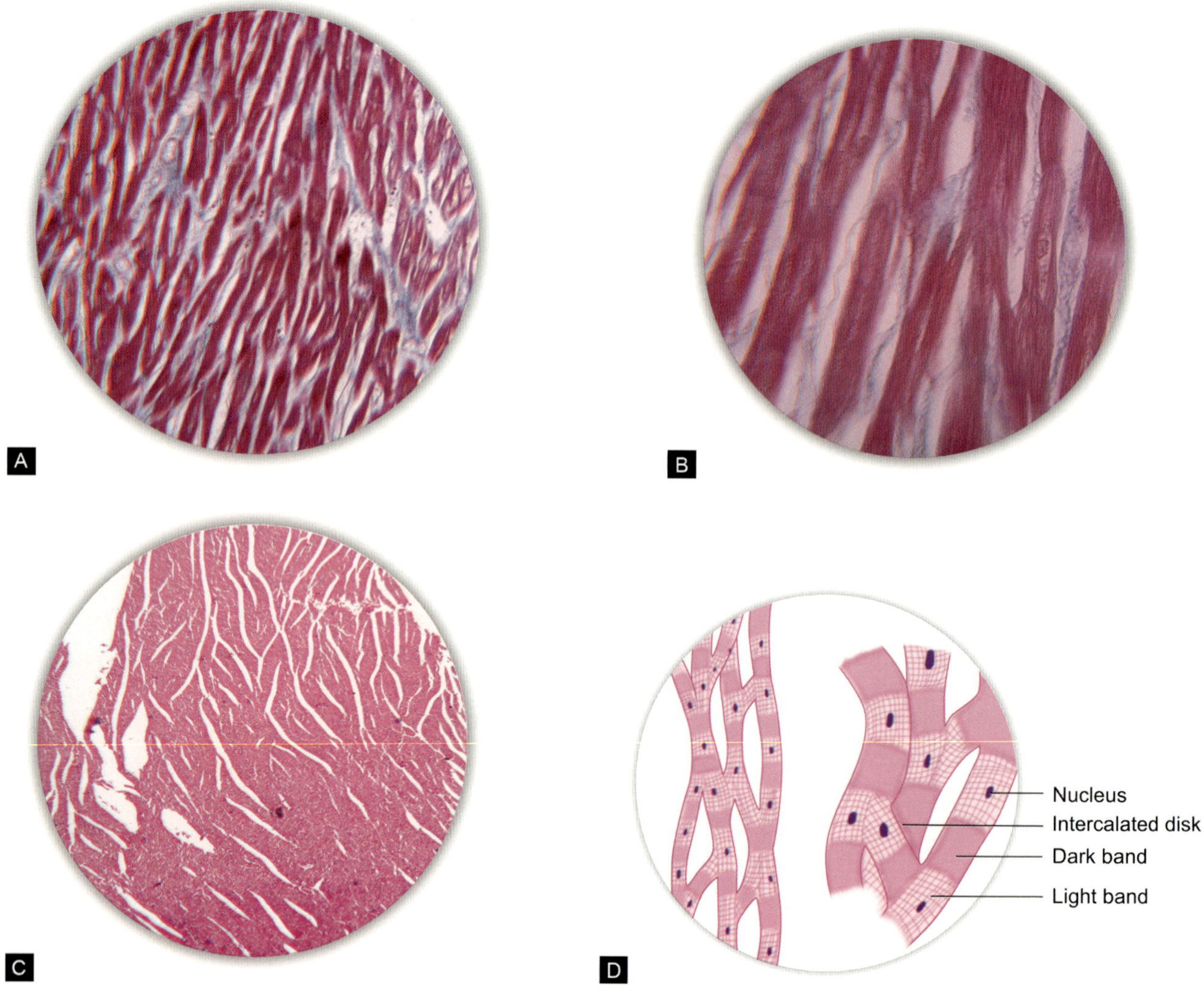

Figures 8.5A to D: Cardiac muscle (Masson's trichrome stain). **A and B.** Photographs; **C.** H&E stain photograph; **D.** Diagrammatic representation (H&E, hematoxylin and Eosin stain) (Note the intercalated disks and nucleus of cardiac muscle).

Clinical Histology

Localized death of cardiac muscle tissue due to the lack of blood supply to that area leads to **myocardial infarction** and it is a case of emergency.

Enlargement of the heart is known as **cardiomegaly** where there is an increased cardiac muscle mass (hypertrophy and hyperplasia) demanding more oxygen for its function. Cardiomegaly is usually secondary to other heart disease like hypertension, valvular defects, rheumatic heart disease, etc.

Discussions

- Where do you see cardiac muscle? How is it different from other muscles in the body?
- What are the differences between cardiac muscle and smooth muscle?
- List the differences between cardiac muscle and skeletal muscle.
- What is an intercalated disk? What is its function?
- Why is heart said to be a functional syncytium?
- State 'all or none law'. Which type of muscle obeys this law?

CHAPTER

9 Nervous Tissue

INTRODUCTION

- Nervous tissue is the highly sophisticated and most complicated tissue, made up of a specialized cell called **neuron.**
- Each and every activity of the cell, tissue and organ in the body is under the control of nervous tissue either directly or indirectly.

CHARACTERISTIC FEATURES

- Nervous tissue is purely **ectodermal** in origin.
- The structural and functional unit of nervous tissue is called **neuron (nerve cell)** and in central nervous system (CNS), neurons are supported by other type of cells called **neuroglial** cells.
- Cytoplasm of the nerve cell is called **axoplasm** and is covered by a tubular sheath called **axolemma.** Both axoplasm and axolemma together form the axis cylinder of nerve fiber.
- A mature neuron has no capacity of regeneration, hence if a part of neuron tissue is lost, it is lost forever.

Neuron

- Neuron is the structural and functional unit of nervous system.
- It is a long slender cylindrical structure with many projections on either side of its tip.
- Based on its morphology and functional capacity, neuron is classified into many types as given in Figure 9.1.

Structure

A typical neuron (Fig. 9.2) has a head part called **cyton** and a long body part called **axon.** It can be explained in detail as follows.

Cyton

- Cyton is also called **cell body, soma** or **perikaryon.**

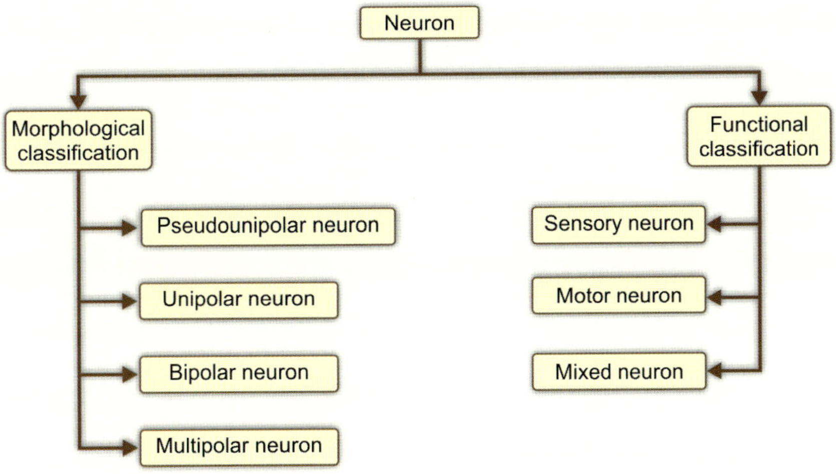

Figure 9.1: Classification of neuron

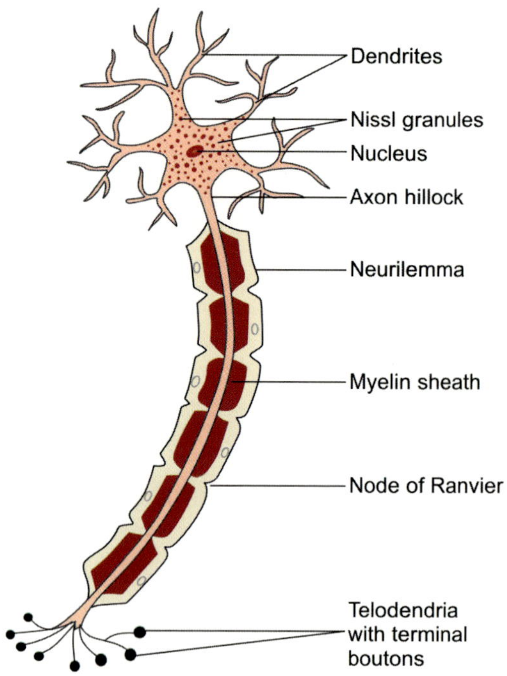

Figure 9.2: Neuron

- Cyton is made up of a prominent nucleus with a nucleolus in it and is surrounded by the cytoplasm.
- Cytoplasm of neuron is rich in neurofibrils, mitochondria, Golgi complex and lysosomes.
- It also contains few characteristic granular structures, which take basic dyes and are called as **Nissl granules (bodies).**
- Nissl granules are nothing but the aggregations of rough endoplasmic reticulum of the cell, which synthesize the proteins required for neurotransmitters and enzyme production.

Dendrites

- Dendrites are the cytoplasmic extensions of the cell body, which highly divide and merges, with the axon terminals (telodendrites) of previous neurons thus forming synapses. They are also supported by neuroglial cells.

Axon

- Axon is one of the longer cytoplasmic extensions of cell body, which runs far away from the cyton.
- **Axon hillock** is the junction where cyton is differentiated into axon.
- Axons are surrounded by a special type of cells called **Schwann cells.**
- These cells secrete **phospholipids,** which encircle around the axon forming **myelin sheath.** Myelin sheath surrounding axon acts like an insulator and helps in conduction of nerve impulses more faster.
- In between the two Schwann cells there is a small interval space, which appears like a node and is called **node of Ranvier.**
- Just above the myelin sheath there is an additional sheath or membrane like structure called **neurilemma.** As it is nothing but the layer of Schwann cell cytoplasm, it is also called **Schwann cell sheath.**

Axon terminals

- This is the terminal part of axon, which is not enclosed by the myelin sheath and it divides into numerous branches called **telodendria** and each telodendria ends with a small swelling called **terminal boutons.**
- Here telodendrites of the axon merge with the dendrites of next neurons and are also supported by neuroglial cells.

Function

The main function of neuron is conduction of nerve impulses. It is always the dendrites, which receive the nerve impulses from previous telodendrites. The nerve impulse travels through cyton and axon finally reaching the telodendrites, which transfer the same nerve impulses to the dendrites of next neuron cell. Hence, the process continues:

- The process of jumping of impulses from one node of Ranvier to another is called saltatory conduction.

Neuroglia

- Neuroglia are the modified connective tissue cells of the CNS, which fill the gap between two neurons.
- Even though they are distributed all over the nervous tissue, they are found predominantly near dendrites and telodendrites of the neuron.

Different types of neuroglia are as follows.

Astrocyte

Astrocytes are the large star-shaped neuroglial cells present in the different parts of brain. They are of two types:

- Fibrous astrocyte.
- Protoplasmic astrocyte.

Fibrous astrocytes: They are the large neuroglial cells with long slender processes. The cytoplasm of the cell is organelle free and it contains an oval nucleus and few fibrillar structures in it. They are predominantly seen in **white matter** of brain.

Protoplasmic astrocytes: They are also large neuroglial cells, but they bear short thick processes with an oval nucleus and few granular structures in its cytoplasm. They are predominantly seen in **grey matter** of brain.

Functions

- Fibrous astrocytes are seen in close contact with the blood capillaries and they form a protective **blood-brain barrier system.**
- Granular astrocytes are seen in between the neurons and they provide support to neurons.

Oligodendrocytes

Oligodendrocytes are the small cells with very few, thin, short processes without excessive branching. They are seen in spinal cord and brain (predominately found in **white matter**).

Functions

Oligodendrocytes act like Schwann cells of peripheral nervous system and help in myelination of nerves of CNS.

Microglia

Microglia are the small glial cells migrated from blood and often called **macrophages of CNS.** They are distributed all over the **grey** and **white matter** of brain.

Functions

Microglia are activated during the inflammation of nerve cells, they become enlarged and migrate to the site of inflammation and phagocytose the infectious agent.

Ependymal Cells

Ependym is the modified simple low columnar or cuboidal epithelium lining the ventricles of brain including the central canal of the spinal cord. They lack the basement membrane and believed to have stereocilia on their surface.

Functions

The cilia of the cells help in absorption of cerebrospinal fluid (CSF) in brain and spinal cord.

PERIPHERAL NERVE (LS)

Slide No. 12

Identification Points

- Long cylindrical nerve fibers
- Central axon with myelin sheath
- Nodes of Ranvier.

a. A longitudinal section (LS) of peripheral nerve (Figs 9.3A and B) shows long cylindrical nerve cells covered by myelin sheath, prominent oval nucleus of Schwann cells and distinct nodes of Ranvier.

Clinical Histology
Inflammation of the neuron associated with degenerative changes of the nerve cell is called **neuritis**
Schwannoma or **Neurilemmoma** is a benign tumor arising from the Schwann cells of cranial and spinal nerve root
Neurofibroma is the most common benign tumor of the peripheral nerve arising from its myelin sheath and is rich in fibrous elements

b. The structure of nerve cell is explained in detail in previous discussions.

Discussions

- What is a neuron? Name different parts of it.
- What are Nissl granules?

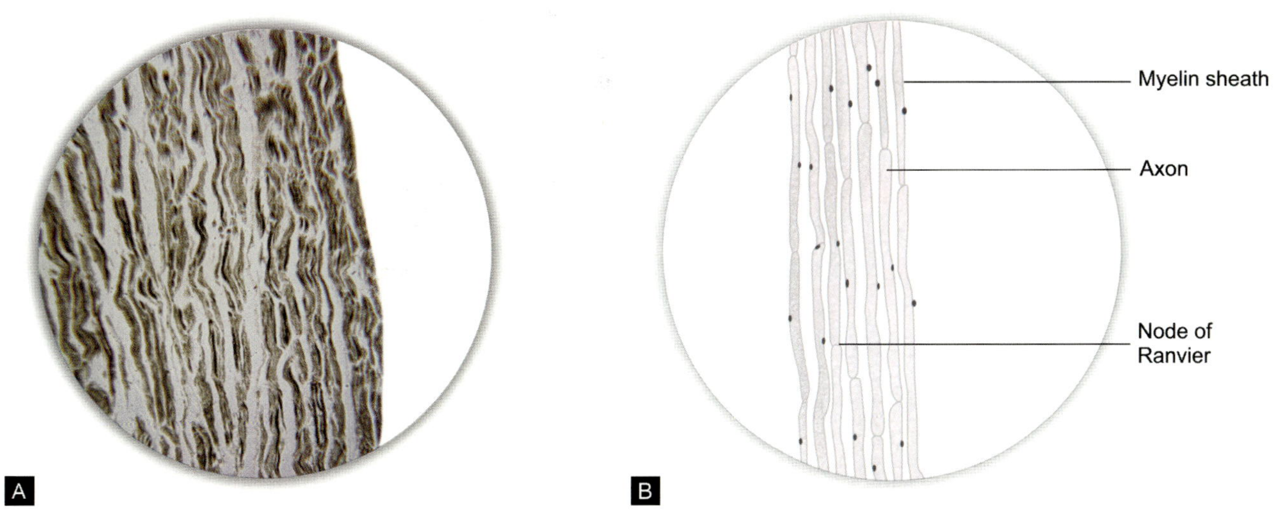

Figures 9.3A and B: Peripheral nerve [longitudinal section (LS)]. **A.** Photograph; **B.** Diagrammatic representation.

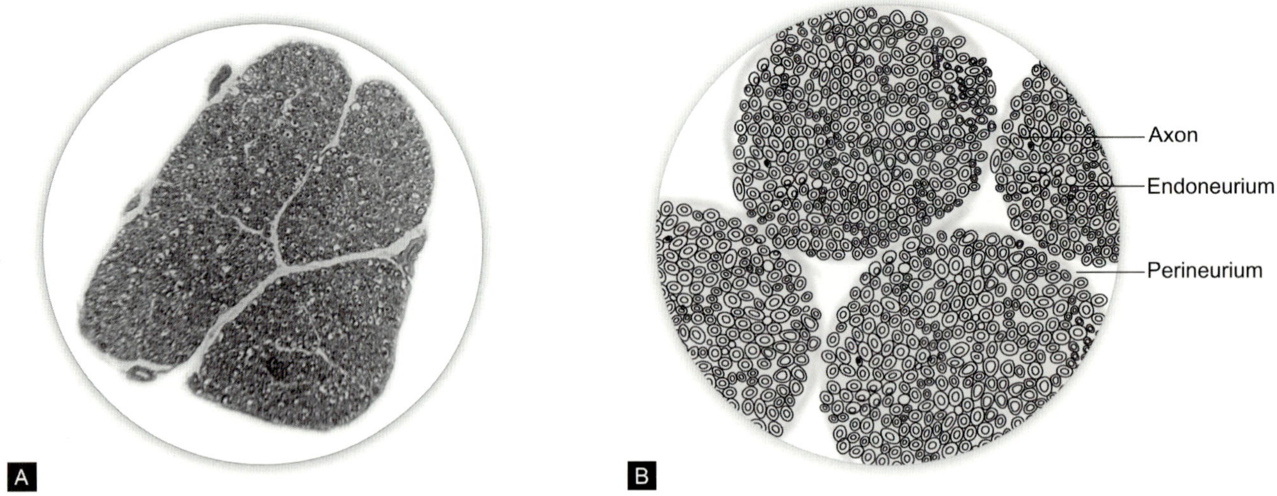

Figures 9.4A and B: Peripheral nerve [transverse sections (TS)]. **A.** Photograph; **B.** Diagrammatic representation.

- How do you differentiate the cyton from axon?
- What are dendrites? What are their functions?
- What are Schwann cells? What is their function?
- What are telodendrites? What is their function?
- What is node of Ranvier?
- What are neuroglia? Name different types of neuroglias with one function each.
- What is saltatory conduction of nerve impulse? Which type of nerve cells exhibit this feature?
- What is neuritis?
- Name two benign tumors of nerve cell.

PERIPHERAL NERVE (TS)

Slide No. 13

Identification Points

- Nerve fibers arranged in fascicles
- Perineurium covering the fascicles
- Epineurium covering the whole nerve.

A transverse section (TS) of peripheral nerve (Figs 9.4A and B) shows following structural features.

Endoneurium

Endoneurium is a loose connective tissue composed of reticular fibers and endoneurial fluid, found surrounding the individual nerve fibers.

Perineurium

Perineurium is a layer of modified fibroblasts and collagen fibers that surrounds the bundle of nerve fibers.

Epineurium

Epineurium is the outermost dense connective tissue sheath surrounding the whole nerve. Sometimes, it is associated with few adipocytes around it, which gives cushion to it.

Discussions

- What is an endoneurium?
- What is a perineurium?
- What is an epineurium?

Ganglion

- Aggregations of cell bodies of neurons outside the central nervous system is called **ganglion.**
- There are two types of ganglia and they are spinal ganglia (sensory) and sympathetic (autonomic) ganglia. The differences between the two are given in Table 9.1.

Table 9.1: Differences between spinal and sympathetic ganglion

Spinal ganglion	Sympathetic ganglion
Capsule is thick	Capsule is thin
Consists of pseudounipolar neurons	Consists of multipolar neurons
Has central nucleus	Has eccentrically placed nucleus
Satellite cells are well-defined	Satellite cells are poorly-defined
Found in groups	Found scattered

SPINAL GANGLION

Slide No. 14

Identification Points

- Large pseudounipolar neurons
- Neurons with centrally placed nuclei
- Well-described satellite cells.

Note: Observe the differences between the cells of spinal ganglion and sympathetic ganglion.

Introduction

Spinal ganglion (Figs 9.5, 9.7A, 9.8A) is the aggregation of neurons in dorsal (posterior) nerve root of spinal cord, therefore, it is also called **dorsal root ganglion.** They are also found in relation to V, VII, IX and X cranial nerves.

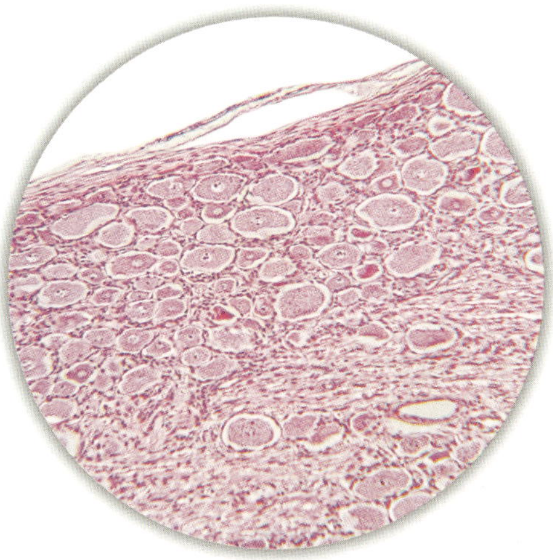

Figure 9.5: Spinal ganglion (photograph)

Structure

It can be explained under following headings.

Capsule

- Each spinal ganglion is covered by a thick capsule made up of dense irregular connective tissue and few blood vessels in it. Usually, capsule merges with the connective tissue of the spinal nerve and epineurium.

Neurons

- A huge number of **pseudounipolar neurons** occurring in group form the main bulk of the ganglion.
- Here each group of neurons is separated from another group of neurons by bundles of **myelinated nerve fiber.**
- Typically, a pseudounipolar neuron is a round to oval in shape having a centrally placed nucleus with a prominent nucleolus.
- Sometimes, cytoplasm of the neuron may contain little brownish lipofuscin pigment in it.
- Here cell body of the neuron is covered by a layer of flattened cells called **satellite cells.**
- Satellite cells present in spinal ganglion are more in number and well-defined than the satellite cells of the sympathetic ganglion. In between two pseudounipolar nerves there exists a connective tissue rich in fibrocytes.

Discussions

- What is a ganglion?
- Name two different types of ganglion?
- What is spinal ganglion? Why it is also called dorsal root ganglion?
- Which type of neurons are seen in a spinal ganglion?
- What are satellite cells?
- Describe the structure of a pseudounipolar neuron of spinal ganglion.

SYMPATHETIC GANGLION

Slide No. 15

Identification Points

- Small multipolar neurons
- Neurons with eccentrically placed nuclei
- Poorly-defined satellite cells.

Structure

A detailed structure of sympathetic (autonomic) ganglion (Figs 9.6, 9.7B, 9.8B) shows followings structures.

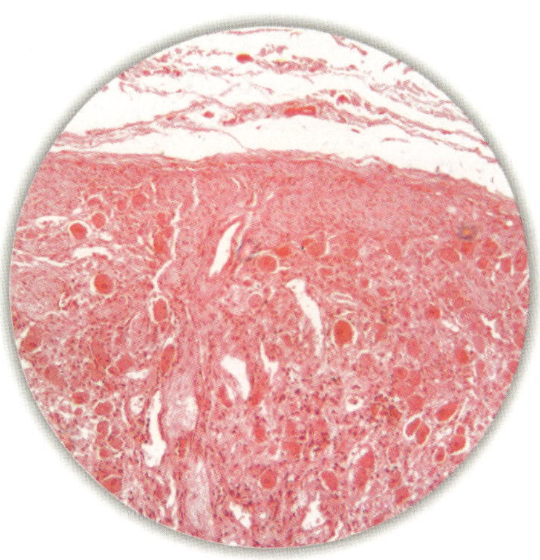

Figure 9.6: Sympathetic ganglion (photograph)

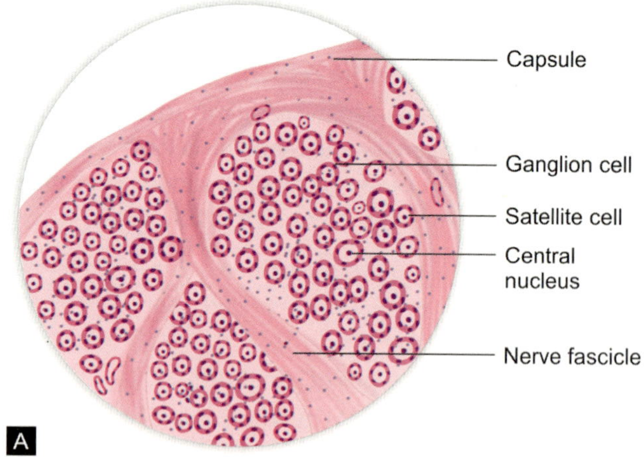

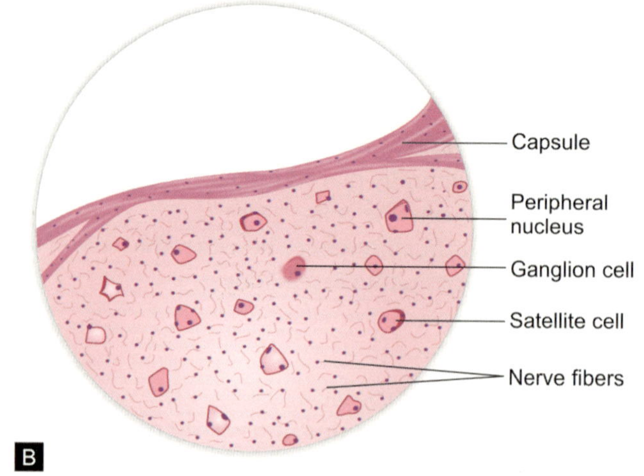

Figures 9.7A and B: Diagrammatic representation of nerve cells. **A.** Spinal ganglion; **B.** Sympathetic ganglion.

Capsule

- Each sympathetic ganglion is covered by a thin capsule made up of dense irregular connective tissue and few blood vessels in it.

Neurons

- Sympathetic ganglion is made up of few numbers of **multipolar neurons** with large amount of connective tissue embedded in the gap. Here multipolar neurons are smaller and scattered here and there within the ganglion.
- Typically, a multipolar neuron is round to oval in shape with an eccentrically placed nucleus in it. Few granules of lipofuscin may also be seen in the cytoplasm of the neuron.

  In this, satellite cells surrounding the multipolar neurons are few in number and are not well-defined.
- Sympathetic ganglion is said to be rich in **non-myelinated nerve fibers,** which are scattered randomly within the ganglion.

Discussions

- What is sympathetic ganglion?
- Which type of neuron is seen in a sympathetic ganglion?
- What are the two important differences between satellite cells of spinal ganglion and that of sympathetic ganglions?
- Describe the structure of a multipolar neuron of sympathetic ganglion.
- Enumerate the differences between spinal ganglions and sympathetic ganglion.

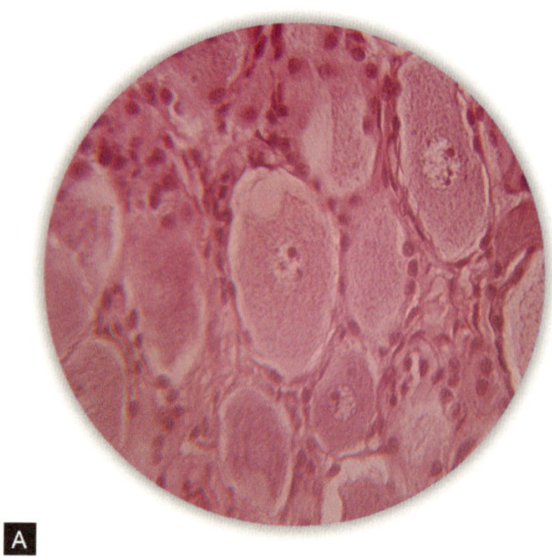

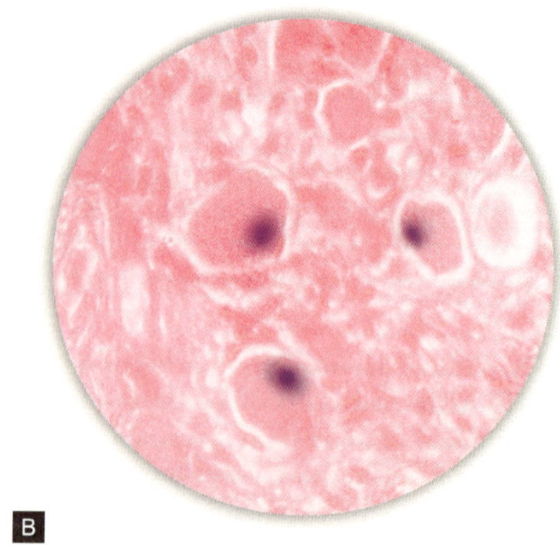

Figures 9.8A and B: Photographs. **A.** Cells of spinal ganglion; **B.** Cells of sympathetic ganglion.

Chapter

10

Lymphoid System

PARTS OF LYMPHOID SYSTEM

Lymphoid system is a part of major defense (system) in the body. It consists of four parts:

- Lymphatic vessels
- Lymph
- Lymphocytes
- Lymphoid organs.

Lymphatic Vessels (Lymphatics)

- Lymphatic vessels arises from the tissue spaces as a delicate network called **lymphatic capillaries.**
- Many lymphatic capillaries unite to form lymphatic vessels, which finally open into heart and circulatory system.
- The largest lymphatic vessel in the body is **thoracic duct,** which drains about 75%–80% of the body. The fluid in the lymphatic vessels is known as **lymph.** Lymphatic vessels contain numerous valves inside them which help in carrying the lymph in same direction.

Lymph

- Lymph (in Latin lympha) is a part of extracellular fluid, which is drained from the interstitial spaces of the tissues.
- Normally lymph is said to be colorless, but because of the presence of fat molecules (chylomicrons) which are absorbed from the small intestine, it appears to be milky white (especially after a heavy fatty meal) hence the lymph is also called **chyle.**
- Lymph is rich in larger protein molecules, fat molecules and lymphocytes.

Lymphocytes

- Lymphocytes are the agranular type of leukocytes (WBC's) produced mainly in bone marrow and other lymphoid organs.
- They are of two types such as T lymphocytes and B lymphocytes.

Further details of lymphocytes will be learnt in the hematopoietic system.

Lymphoid Organs

These are the sites of active proliferation and differentiation of the lymphocytes.

They are of two types:

- Primary lymphoid organs, e.g. thymus, bone marrow.
- Secondary lymphoid organs, e.g. spleen, palatine tonsil, mucosa-associated lymphoid tissue (MALT).

LYMPH NODE

Slide No. 16

Identification Points

- Subcapsular sinus or space
- Cortex showing lymphatic nodules
- Medulla rich in blood vessels.

Introduction

- Lymph node (Figs 10.1A and B) is a bean-shaped structure, widely distributed in the path of lymphatic vessels. The size of the lymph node varies from small pinhead up to bead or shelled almond. They are also called **lymph glands or lymphatic nodes.**

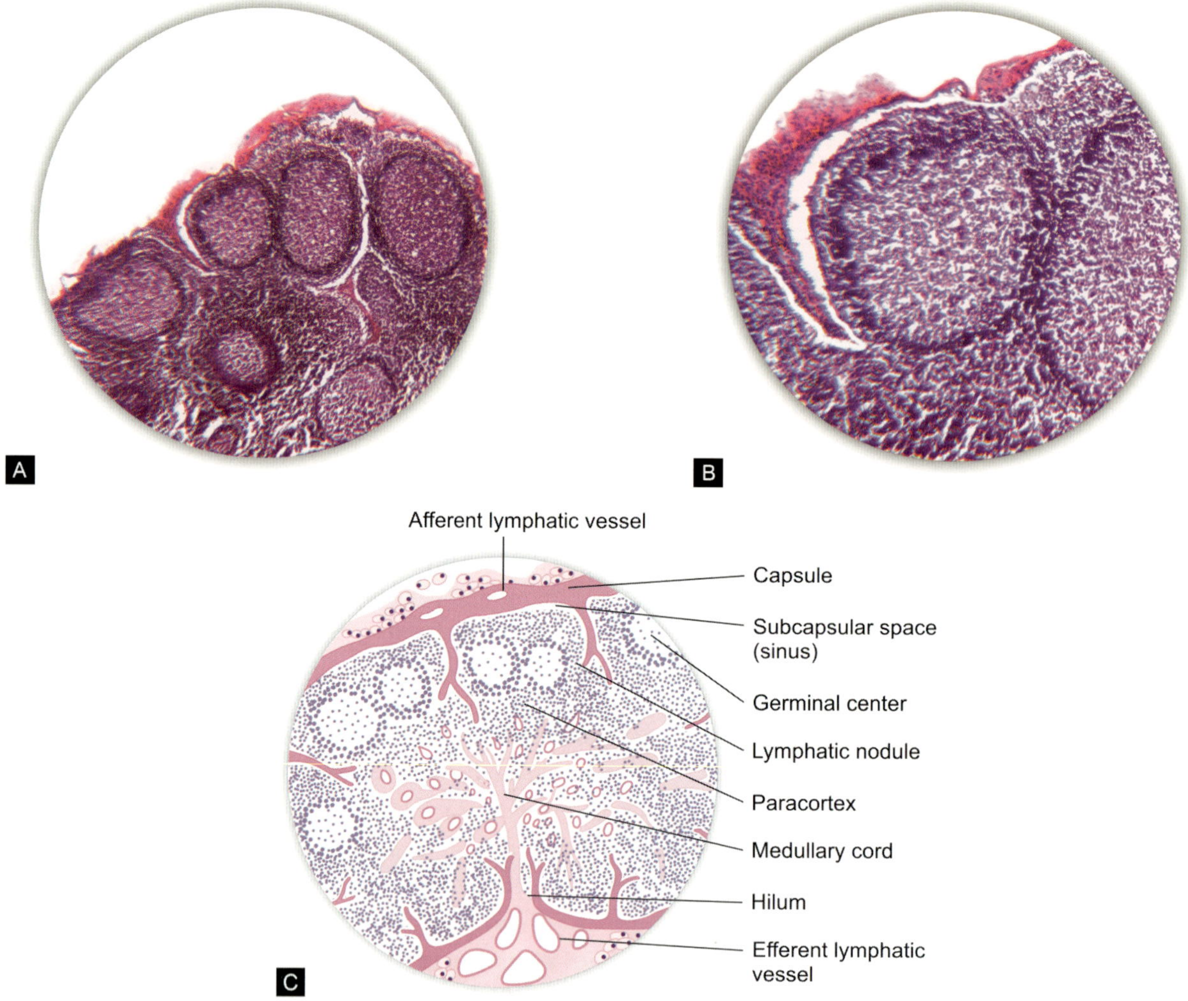

Figures 10.1A to C: Lymph node. **A.** Photograph; **B.** Highly magnified view of lymph node showing subcapsular sinus; **C.** Diagrammatic representation.

- It has got two surfaces, i.e. convex surface, where many afferent lymphatic vessels enter the cortex through the capsule and a concave surface (hilus), where usually one or two efferent lymphatic vessels leave the medulla through capsule.

Structure

Structure of a typical lymph node shows following parts.

Capsule: It is an outermost, protective covering of lymph node, made up of dense irregular connective tissue rich in collagen fibers and few elastic fibers:

- Many septae (trabeculae) arise from the connective tissue capsule and divide the lymph node into many lobules, and they carry the blood vessels along their course. Just below the connective tissue capsule there is a minute space or gap called **subcapsular sinus** (Fig. 10.1C).
- Afferent lymphatic vessels penetrate the capsule and open into the subcapsular sinus, these sinuses extend into the lymph node along the trabeculae forming **trabecular sinus.** These become continuous with the **medullary sinus** and finally open into the efferent lymphatic vessels near the hilum.

Cortex: It is an outer part of the lymph node, which is more darkly stained than inner part (medulla). It consists of many rounded structures called **lymphatic nodules:**

- Lymphatic nodule is a ring like structure with lightly stained central area called **germinal center** and darkly stained outer area.
- Germinal center is an active site, which produces immature B lymphocytes called **lympho-blasts.** They are arranged loosely with lightly stained nuclei; hence the germinal center appears to be lighter.

- As the B lymphocytes move to the periphery they become matured and more compactly arranged with darkly stained nuclei; hence the outer area appears darker than the inner germinal center
- Lymphatic nodules are surrounded by few other types of cells like macrophages, plasma cells, reticular cells, etc.
- The deeper part of the cortex is known as **para cortex,** which is **thymus dependent** zone and mainly consists of T lymphocytes with the absence of lymphatic nodules.

Medulla: It is an inner part of the lymph node, which is lightly stained rather than cortex. It contains many branching and anastomosing cords of lymphocytes, plasma cells and few macrophages forming medullary cords. In between two medullary cords numerous medullary sinuses are seen. Medulla is rich in blood capillaries.

Functions

- Acts as active center of lymphocyte production.
- Filters the lymph.
- Acts as the center of phagocytosis by trapping the foreign antigens.
- It idirectly helps in giving immunity to the body by producing lymphocytes.

Clinical Histology
Inflammation of the lymph node is known as **lymphadenitis**
Small, shrunken and matted lymph nodes are seen in tuberculosis
Metastasis of any cancer occurs mainly through lymph nodes

Discussions

- Describe the size and shape of a lymph node.
- What is hilum and what does it contain?
- What is subcapsular sinus?
- What is lymphatic nodule?
- What is germinal center? What does it contain?
- Which are the different types of cells seen in the cortex, other than lymphocytes?
- Which is the location of B lymphocyte, T lymphocyte in the lymph node?
- What is paracortex? What is its significance?
- What are medullary cords?
- List the functions of lymph node.
- Explain the mode of passage of lymph through the lymph node.
- What is lymphadenitis?

SPLEEN

Slide No. 17

Identification Points

- Outermost capsule with trabeculae
- White pulp with eccentrically placed arteriole
- Red pulp rich in blood sinusoids.

Introduction

- Spleen (Figs 10.2A to C) is the largest lymphoid organ in body located in the left hypochondrium of the abdomen.
- Spleen develops in the **5th week** of intrauterine life. It develops as small nodules of **mesenchymal cells** derived from the mesogastrium and later the entire nodules fuse to form spleen.

Structure

Structure can be explained under the following headings:

- Capsule
- Stroma
- Parenchyma.

Capsule: It is an outermost protective covering made up of dense irregular connective tissue with few smooth muscles fibers in it:

- Capsule sends many septae into the parenchyma, which divide the spleen into many smaller divisions. They also carry the blood vessels along with them.

Stroma: It consists of an extracellular matrix with a delicate network of reticular fibers supporting the parenchyma. It also contains fibroblasts (reticular cells) and few macrophages in it.

Parenchyma: The spleen shows mainly two regions:

White pulp: Splenic artery after entering into the hilum of spleen divides into five branches. Each branch undergoes further subdivisions as it travels through the trabecular network and enters the intertrabecular space as **central artery:**

- Here it is covered by a dense sheath of lymphocytes forming a ring like structure and is called **white pulp**
- At some places white pulp becomes more thicker than elsewhere containing lymphatic nodule like structures in it and are called **malpighian bodies** they can be easily differentiated from lymphatic nodules of the lymph node by looking at the eccentrically placed arteriole in it.

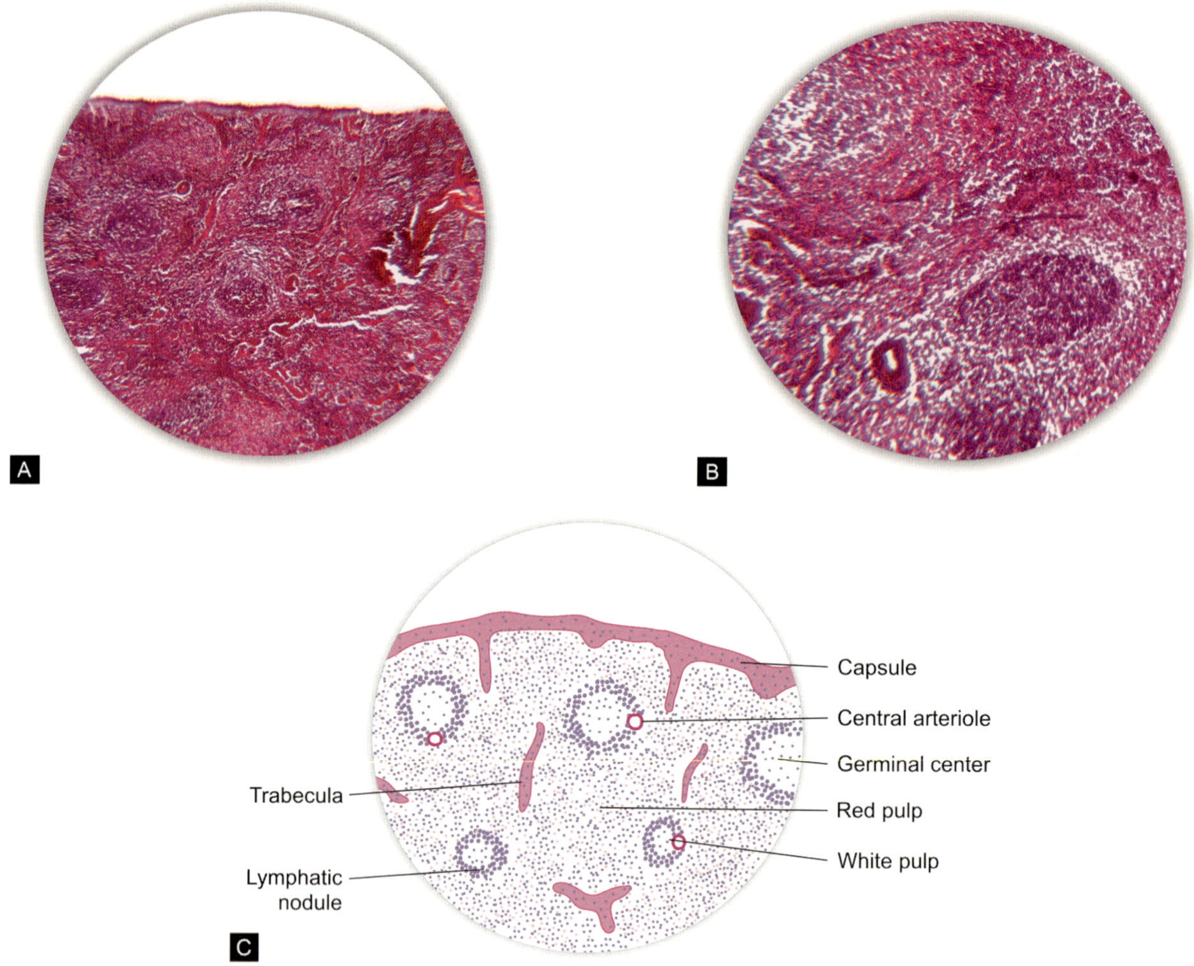

Figures 10.2A to C: Spleen. **A.** Photograph; **B.** Highly magnified view; **C.** Diagrammatic representation (please note the white pulp with eccentric arteriole).

Red pulp: Central artery of the white pulp further divides into many straight arterioles called **penicilli:**

- Each penicillus shows a localized thickening of macrophages around its wall thus decreasing the lumen size forming **ellipsoid arterioles.**
- The distal part of the ellipsoid arterioles are dilated to form **ampulla,** which opens into the reticular framework thus pouring the blood into the reticular framework of the spleen. This part of the parenchyma is called **red pulp.**
- Red pulp is rich in lymphocytes (B and T), macrophages and other blood cells, which appear like cords and they are called **splenic cords of Billroth.**
- The blood from red pulp enters into the sinusoids and is drained by many venules and veins finally come out of the hilum through splenic vein.

Theories of Splenic Circulation

Following theories are put forward to explain the mechanism of blood circulation:

- **Open theory:** According to this theory blood from the arterioles is poured into the splenic cords, which will enter the sinusoids for its further drainage. This type of circulation is seen in red pulp.
- **Closed theory:** According to this theory the blood from the arterioles directly poured into the sinusoids which is drained by the branches of splenic vein. This type of circulation is seen in white pulp.
- **Compromise theory:** This is the most widely accepted theory according to which splenic circulation is combination of both open and close theory of circulation.

Functions

- Spleen is the site of hemopoiesis in fetal life.
- Acts as store-house of blood.
- Acts as part of reticuloendothelial system by destructing the old red blood cells (RBCs).
- Produces lymphocytes, which play an important role in giving immunity.

  Note: In spite of all these functions spleen is not absolutely essential for life, because all these functions can also be performed by other organs in the body like liver, bone, etc.

Clinical Histology
Enlargement of the spleen is known as **splenomegaly** and is seen in malaria, kala-azar and typhoid
Surgical removal of the spleen is termed as **splenectomy**

Discussions

- Which is the largest lymphoid organ in the body?
- What is white pulp?
- What is red pulp?
- What are malpighian bodies? How do you differentiate it from the lymphatic nodules of the lymph node?
- What are splenic cords of Billroth?
- Describe the splenic circulation.
- Name the different theories put forward to explain the splenic circulation.
- Which is the most accepted theory of splenic circulation? Why?
- Enumerate the functions of spleen.
- What is splenectomy?
- What is splenomegaly?

THYMUS

Slide No. 18

Identification Points

- Outermost capsule with incomplete septae
- Lobules with cortex and medulla
- Hassall's corpuscles in medulla.

Introduction

- Thymus (Figs 10.3A and B) is a primary lymphoid organ situated in the anterior and superior mediastinum of thorax.
- The gland resembles to thymic leaf, an ancient Greek plant hence the name **thymus gland.**
- Thymus develops from the endoderm of third pharyngeal pouch and its lymphocytes are derived from the mesoderm. Hence, the gland is also known as **lymphoepithelial organ.**
- The size of the gland highly varies with the age of an individual, it is larger in infants and children as the age advances it becomes degenerated and infiltrated by adipose tissue.

Structure

Structure of thymus shows following parts.

Capsule: Like other organs, the capsule of the gland is made up of thin layer of dense irregular connective tissue rich in collagen and elastic fibers with fibroblasts.

The connective tissue septae arising from the capsule divide the glandular parenchyma into many incomplete lobules and they also carry the blood vessels, afferent lymphatics and nerves along their course.

Parenchyma: It is in the form of lobules. A typical lobule shows an inner lighter area called **medulla** and an outer darker area called **cortex.**

Cortex: It is an outer area of lobule rich in densely packed T lymphocytes with prominent nuclei hence the cortex appears darker than the medulla. Cortex also contains few macrophages and epithelioreticular cells.

Medulla: It is an inner area of the lobule with loosely arranged lymphocytes and numerous epithelioreticular cells. Here medulla of one lobule is continuous with another medullary lobules of the gland.

Hassall's corpuscles: These are the rounded eosinophilic bodies with a central homogeneous area of hyalinization surrounded by few concentric layers of flattened epithelial cells. Hassall's corpuscles (Fig. 10.3C) are seen in the medulla of the thymic lobules and their exact function is not known. They are derived from endoderm of third pharyngeal pouch. The number of Hassall's corpuscles is closely related to the age of an individual and their number increases as the age advances.

Blood-thymus barrier: Few cells and epitheliocytes of the thymus become flat and joined to form sheets covering the internal surface of the capsule, septae and the blood vessels, and they act like blood-thymus barrier thus prevent the entry of foreign antigens from the blood in to the thymic tissue.

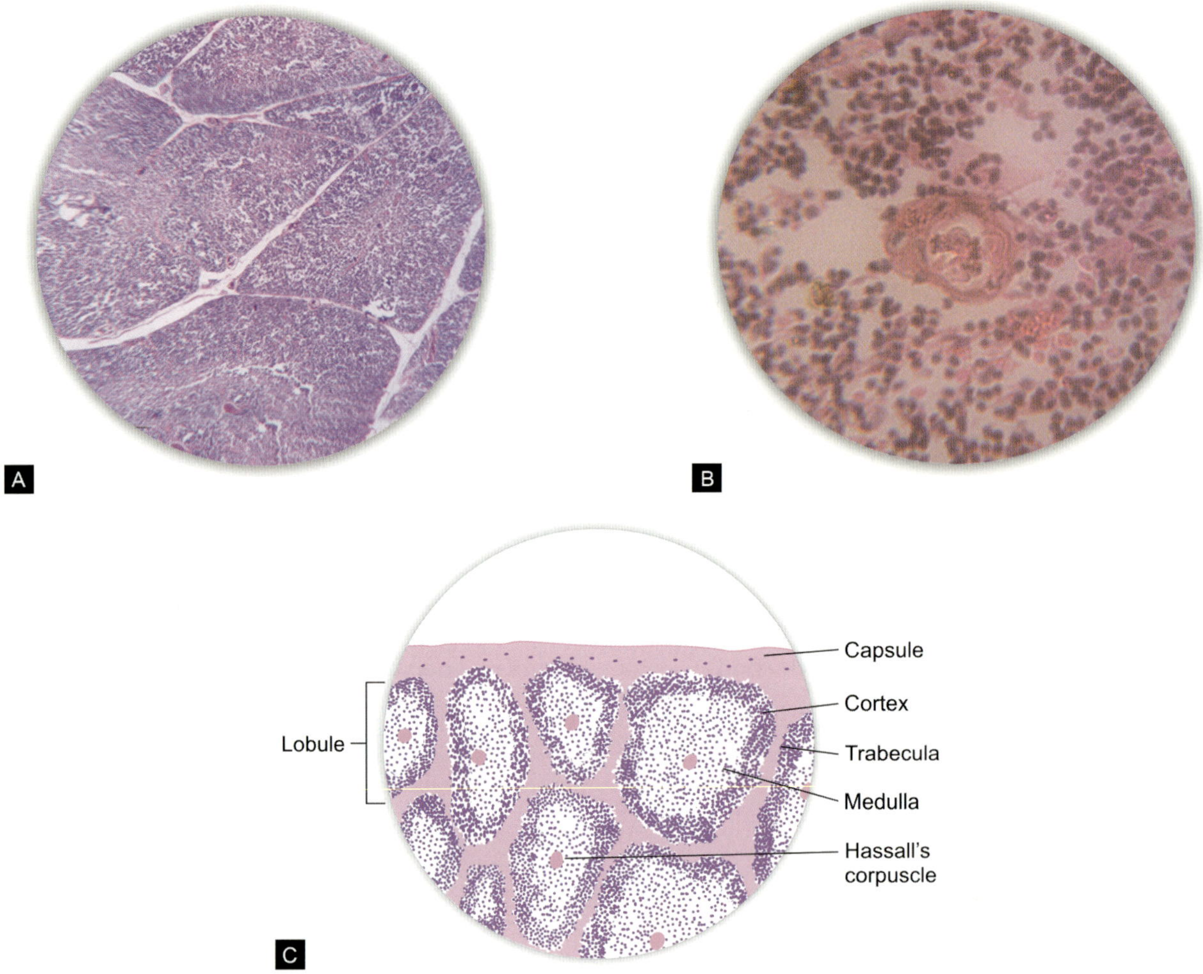

Figures 10.3A to C: Thymus. **A.** Photograph; **B.** Highly magnified view showing Hassall's corpuscle; **C.** Diagrammatic representation.

Functions

- Production and maturation of T lymphocytes.
- Epithelial reticular cells of thymus produces a hormone **thymosin,** which is necessary for the proliferation and maturation of T lymphocytes.

Discussions

- Why is thymus also called lymphoepithelial organ?
- What are epithelioreticular cells? What is their function?
- What are Hassall's corpuscles?

PALATINE TONSIL

Slide No. 19

Identification Points

- Deep tonsillar crypts
- Stratified squamous non-keratinized epithelium lining the surface
- Lymphatic nodules with germinal center.

Introduction

Palatine tonsil (Figs 10.4A and B) is a diffuse mass of lymphoid tissue seen in the lateral wall of the oropharynx in

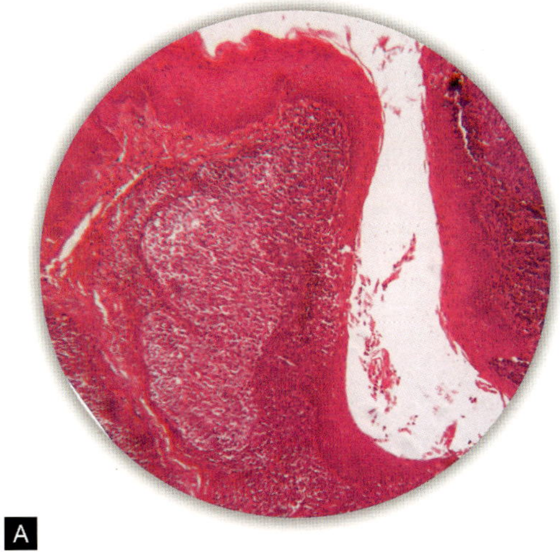

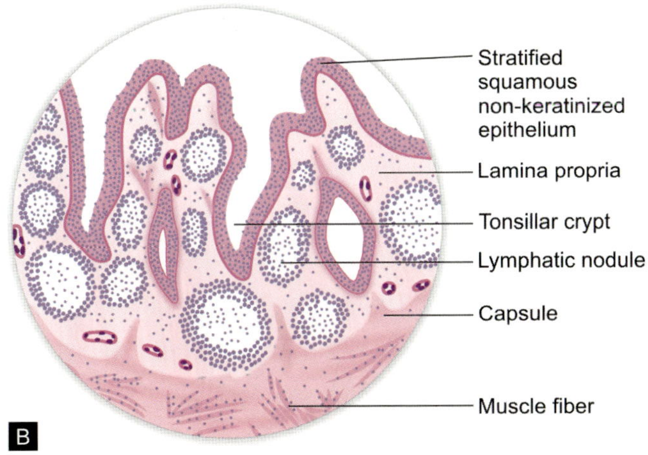

Figures 10.4A and B: Palatine tonsil. **A.** Photograph; **B.** Diagrammatic representation.

the tonsillar fossa. Since it is an almond-shaped structure located near the palate hence it is called **palatine tonsil** (Latin: Tonsilla—almond).

Structure

Structure of palatine tonsil shows the following details.

Surface epithelium: Surface of the tonsil is covered by a layer of stratified squamous non- keratinized epithelium. The surface epithelium dips into the substance of the tonsil forming many crypts called tonsillar crypts. There is a thin layer of connective tissue capsule covering the gland incompletely, which sends septae (trabeculae) with blood vessels and passes toward the surface of tonsil between the lymphatic nodules.

Some mucous glands are also seen near the bottom of crypts, which opens into the tonsillar crypts.

Lymphatic nodules: These are the rounded ring like structures with an inner lighter area made up of immature lymphocytes (lymphoblasts) forming germinal center and outer darkly stained brim of compactly arranged lymphocytes (B and T). Occasionally, some lymphocytes of the tonsil are discharged into the saliva forming **salivary corpuscles.**

Functions

- Produces lymphocytes.
- Protects gastrointestinal and respiratory tract against entry of pathogen.

Clinical Histology
Inflammation of the palatine tonsil is called **tonsillitis**
Surgical removal of the tonsil is called **tonsillectomy**

Discussions

- What is the location of palatine tonsil?
- Name the surface epithelium covering the palatine tonsils.
- What are tonsillar crypts?
- Enumerate the functions of tonsil.
- What are salivary corpuscles?
- What do you mean by the word palatine tonsil?
- What is tonsillitis?
- What is tonsillectomy?

CHAPTER

11 Circulatory System

INTRODUCTION

Heart and blood vessels together form cardiovascular system (Fig. 11.1). Blood vessels include arteries, veins and their derivatives.

Artery: It is a vessel, which carries oxygenated blood. An artery caries blood away from heart.

Vein: It is a vessel, which carries deoxygenated blood. A vein carries blood toward the heart.

Capillary: It is the channel, which connects the arterial system and venous system together.

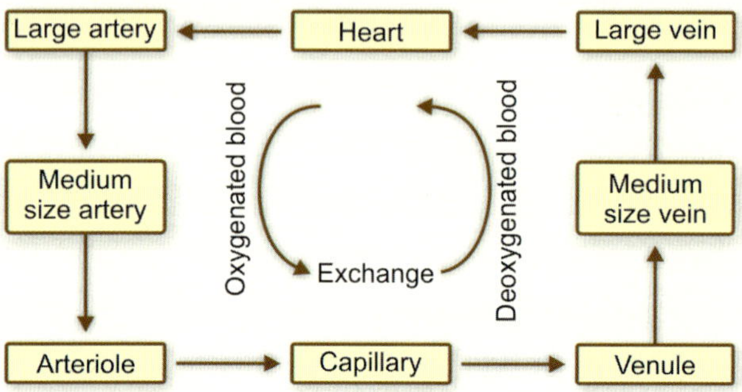

Figure 11.1: Cardiovascular system

GENERAL FEATURES OF A BLOOD VESSEL

Histologically, a typical blood vessel shows three different layers in it (Table 11.1).

Tunica intima: It is the innermost layer of the blood vessel lined by **simple squamous epithelium or endothelium.**

- Just below the endothelium, there is a thin layer of subendothelial connective tissue and **internal elastic lamina,** which is nothing, but a thin streak of elastic fiber.

Tunica media: It is the middle layer of a blood vessel seen just below the tunica intima.

- It is made up of either smooth muscles or elastic fibers
- Tunica media is limited by a thin layer of elastic fibers called '**external elastic lamina**'.

Tunica adventitia: It is an outermost layer of a vessel which is made up of dense irregular connective tissue.

Table 11.1: Different layers of artery and vein

Artery	Vein
Lumen is almost circular	Lumen is collapsed or irregular
Tunica media is larger	Tunica media is smaller
Tunica adventitia is smaller	Tunica adventitia is larger
Carries oxygenated blood	Carries deoxygenated blood

LARGE ARTERY (Figs 11.2A and B)

Slide No. 20

Identification Points

- Circular lumen
- Thick tunica media rich in elastic fibers
- Vasa vasorum in tunica adventitia.

Introduction

- An artery is the one, which carries oxygenated blood in it. Usually, thickness of large sized arterial wall is less than its lumen diameter. A large sized artery is rich in elastic fibers in it hence it is also named as **elastic artery,** e.g. aorta, axillary artery, subclavian artery, iliac artery.

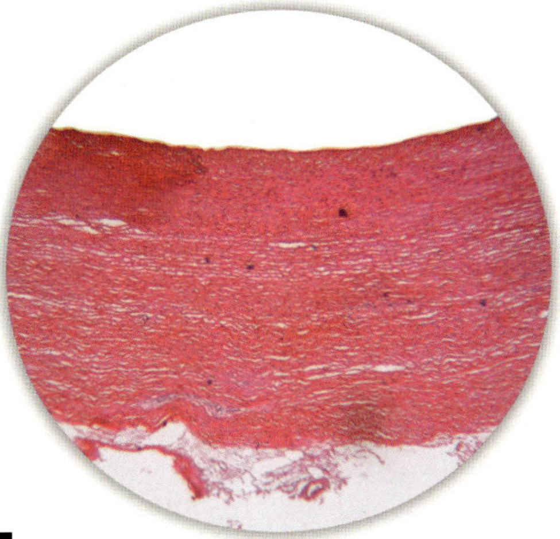
A

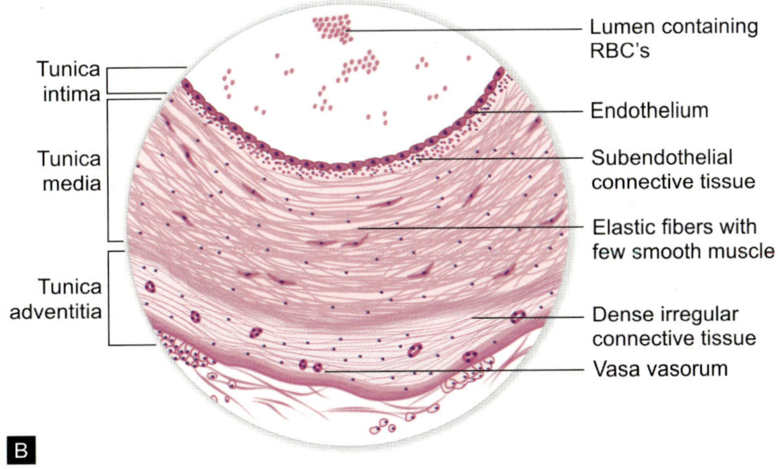

B

Figures 11.2A and B: Large artery. **A.** Photograph; **B.** Diagrammatic representation.

Structure

Structure of an elastic artery can be explained as follows.

Tunica intima: It is the innermost layer of a vessel lined by simple squamous epithelium also called **endothelium.** Here all the cells are single layered and are resting on the basement membrane:

- Just below the basement membrane there is a thin layer of subendothelial connective tissue along with an internal elastic lamina.

Tunica media: It is the middle layer of a vessel, which is larger than other two layers:

- Here it is rich in bundles of elastic fibers with few smooth cells in it here and there.
- Internal and external elastic lamina are present in large sized artery, but still it cannot be differentiated because of huge amount of elastic fibers in the tunica media.

Tunica adventitia: It is the outermost layer of the vessel made up of dense irregular connective tissue:

- In an artery, tunica adventitia layer is smaller than the tunica medial layer.
- There are many small vessels in the adventitia layer of large sized artery and those are called **vasa vasorum.**
- Since the thickness of a large sized artery is larger, the adventitial layer fails to get its nutrition from intimal layer by simple diffusion. Thus vasa vasorum plays an important role in nourishing the tunica adventitia and tunica media layer.

Functions

- Endothelial layer lining the tunica intima is antithrombotic and nutritive in function.
- Elastic fibers of the tunica media expand the arterial wall thus helps in maintaining normal arterial pressure and blood flow.
- Connective tissue layer of the tunica adventitia prevents undue stretching and rupture of the artery.

Clinical Histology
Inflammation of the artery is known as **arteritis.**
Atherosclerosis is characterized by the formation. Atheromatic plaque in the tunica intima of larger blood vessels reducing its lumen size.
Endothelial lining of an artery is antithrombotic in nature. Any breach or discontinuity in its layer leads to the formation of thrombus, which, in turn, may lead to **myocardial infarction** or **heart attack.**
An abnormal and permanent dilatation of an artery is called **aneurysm** and is more common in large sized arteries like aorta.

Discussions

- Name few large-sized arteries.
- Why large-sized artery is also called elastic artery?
- List the different layers of an artery.
- List the differences between an artery and a vein.
- Which layer of a large-sized artery is rich in elastic fibers?
- Why internal and external elastic laminas are not seen clearly in large-sized artery?

- What is vasa vasorum? What is its function?
- Which layer of an artery is antithrombotic in nature?
- Enumerate the functions of each layer in an elastic artery.
- Define atherosclerosis.
- What is aneurysm?

MEDIUM SIZE ARTERY (Figs 11.3A and B)

Slide No. 21

Identification Points

- Circular lumen
- Prominent internal elastic lamina
- Tunica media rich in circular smooth muscles.

Introduction

- An artery where thickness of its wall is almost equal to its diameter of lumen is called medium-sized artery.
- Medium-sized artery is rich in smooth muscle fibers, hence the name given **muscular artery, e.g.** brachial artery, radial artery, ulnar artery, popliteal artery, etc.

Structure

Structure of an muscular artery can be explained as follows.

Tunica intima: It is the inner-most layer made up of endothelium. A thin layer of subendothelial connective tissue is seen beneath the endothelial lining with a prominent internal elastic lamina.

Tunic media: It is the middle layer of an artery with a large number of smooth muscle fibers in it. Here few long wavy collagen fibers are also seen between the muscle cells with a prominent external elastic lamina.

Tunica adventitia: It is the outermost layer made up of dense irregular connective tissue. Vasa vasorum are absent in this layer since it can be easily nourished by simple diffusion of the nutrients up to this layer.

Functions

- Tunica intima is antithrombotic in function.
- Muscle layers of tunica media contracts thus pushing the blood toward smaller blood vessels and tissues.
- Tunica adventitia is supportive and protective in function.

Clinical Histology

Monckeberg's medial sclerosis is a peripheral vascular disease characterized by the deposition of calcium in the tunica media of medium-sized blood vessels. Other peripheral vascular diseases are Buerger's disease, Raynaud's disease, Alzheimer's disease, etc.

Arteriole (Figs 11.4A and B)

- Arteriole is a small blood vessel with less than 1 mm in diameter.
- An arteriole is made up of single layer of endothelium with few muscle fibers around it. It lacks internal elastic lamina in it.

Capillary (Figs 11.5A and B)

- Capillary is a minute microvasculature with a diameter of 8–10 micron.

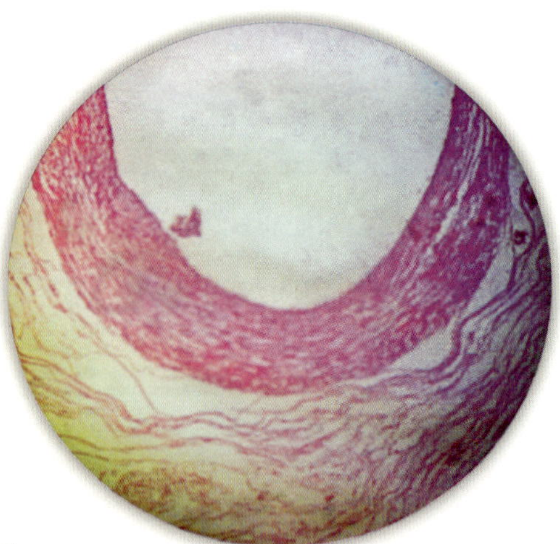

A

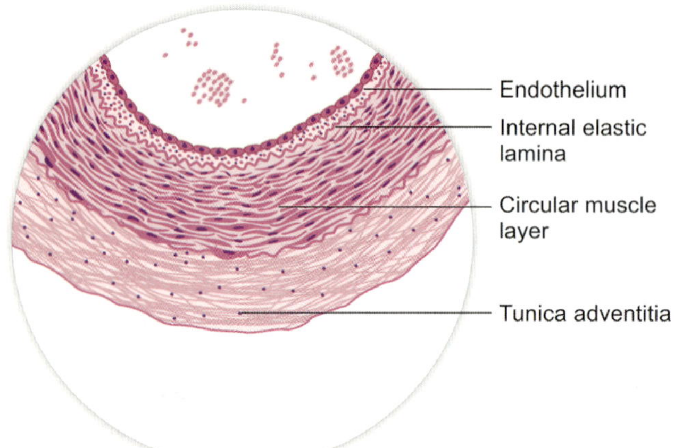

B

Figures 11.3A and B: Medium size artery. **A.** Photograph; **B.** Diagrammatic representation.

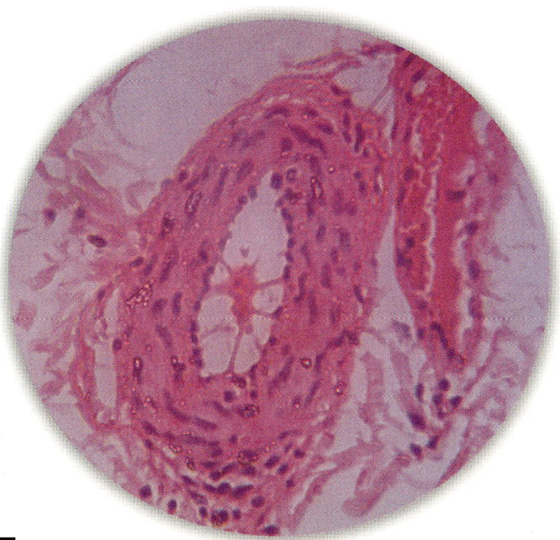

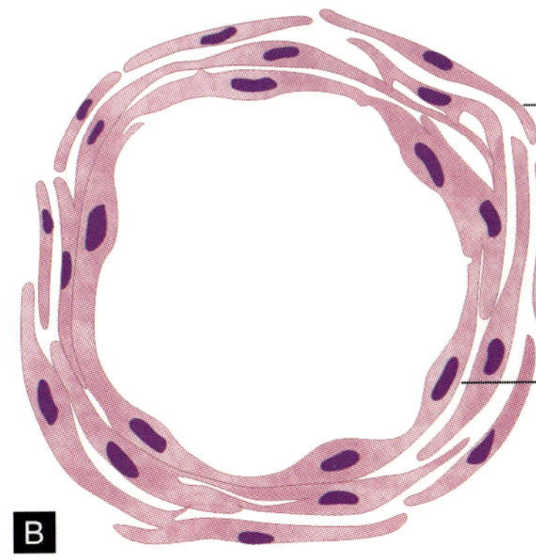

Figures 11.4A and B: Arteriole. **A.** Photograph; **B.** Diagrammatic representation.

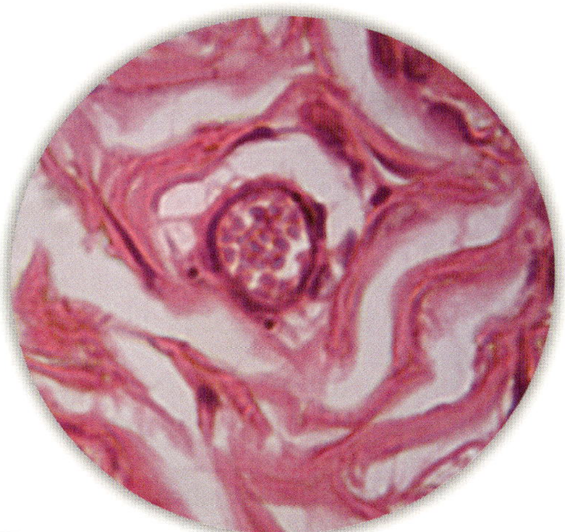

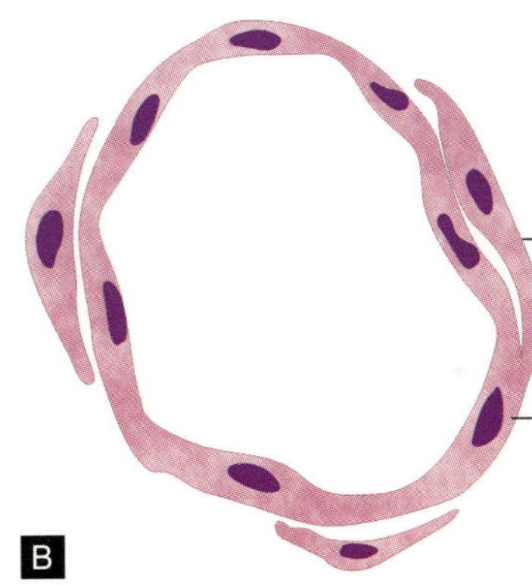

Figures 11.5A and B: Capillary. **A.** Photograph; **B.** Diagrammatic representation.

- It is made up of an inner endothelium layer lined upon a glycoprotein layer called **basal lamina.** A cell surrounding the capillary may be seen, which acts like a muscle cell and is called **pericyte.**

LARGE SIZE VEIN (Figs 11.6A and B)

Slide No. 22

Identification Points

- Collapsed lumen
- Thin tunica media with circular muscle fibers
- Thick tunica adventitia with longitudinal smooth muscles and vasa vasorum.

Introduction

- A vein is a vessel, which carries deoxygenated blood in it.
- Superior vena cava and inferior vena cava are the large sized vein present in the body.

Structure

A detailed structure of a large vein can be explained as follows.

Tunica intima: It is the inner-most layer of vein consisting of endothelial lining with a delicate framework of subendothelial connective tissue underneath it. Here internal elastic lamina is poorly defined.

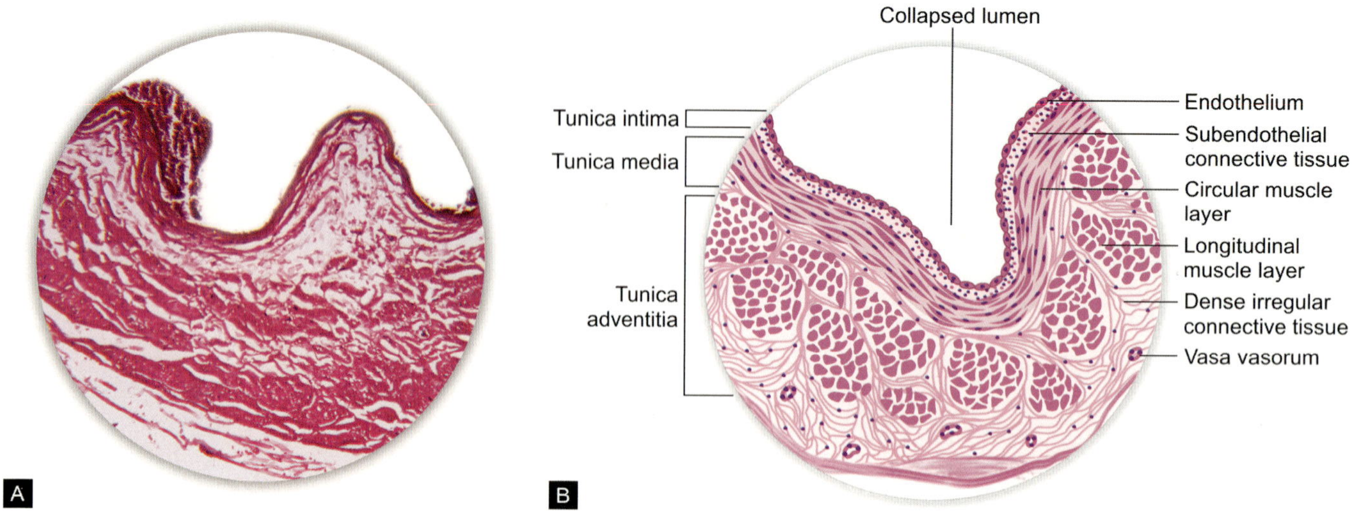

Figures 11.6A and B: Large size vein. **A.** Photograph; **B.** Diagrammatic representation.

Tunica media: It is the middle layer, which is usually very thin with few circular smooth muscles in it. Here also external elastic lamina is not properly visible.

Tunica adventitia: It is the outermost thick layer of vein made up of many bundles of longitudinal muscle fibers and dense irregular connective tissue. Tunica adventitia of large vein contains **vasa vasorum,** which helps in nourishing the adventitial layer.

Functions

- Endothelial layer of tunica intima is antithrombotic and nutritive in function.
- Smooth muscles of tunica media aid the contraction of the vein.
- Thick layer of longitudinal muscle cells powerfully contract and push the deoxygenated blood toward the heart whereas dense irregular connective tissue is supportive and protective in function.

Discussions

- What is a vein ?
- Name the differences between an artery and a vein.
- Name the layers of large vein.
- Which layer is thicker in large vein?
- List the functions of different layers of a large vein.
- List the histological differences between large-sized artery and large-sized vein.

MEDIUM SIZE VEIN (Figs 11.7A and B)

Slide No. 23

Identification Points

- Collapsed lumen
- Tunica media containing circular smooth muscles
- Tunica adventitia with dense irregular connective tissue.

Introduction

- A medium-sized vein is rich in numerous valves, which facilitate the flow of blood only in one direction, **e.g.** popliteal vein, axillary vein, internal jugular vein, basilic vein, cephalic vein, etc.

Structure

A detailed structure of a medium size vein can be explained as follows.

Tunica intima: It is lined by single layer of simple squamous epithelium and also called **endothelium.** There is a small layer of subendothelial connective tissue with the lack of internal elastic lamina in it.

Tunica media: It is the middle layer, which is thinner as compared to the tunica media of medium-sized artery. It contains few layers of circular smooth muscle fibers supported by connective tissue, which mainly contains collagen fibers in it.

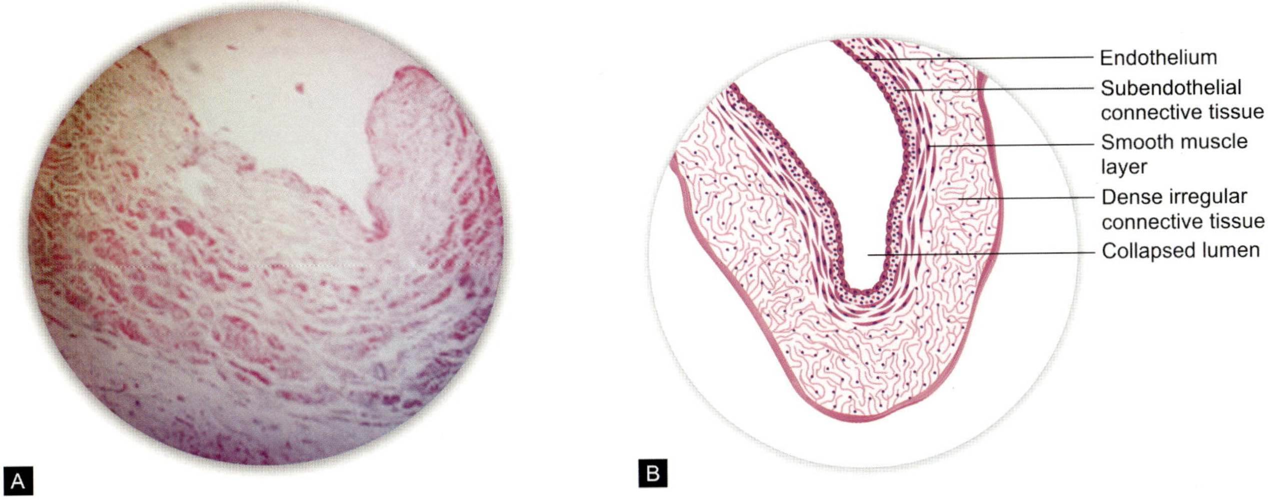

Figures 11.7A and B: Medium size vein. **A.** Photograph; **B.** Diagrammatic representation.

Tunica adventitia: It is an outermost layer made up of dense irregular connective tissue with the absence of vasa vasorum.

Valve: It is the extension of tunica intimal layer in the lumen of vein. It is lined by an endothelium with little subendothelial connective tissue underneath it. It allows the flow of blood only in one direction.

Clinical Histology

Abnormally dilated and tortuous veins are called **varicose veins:**
- It is most commonly seen in medium- and small-sized veins of the lower limb
- Varicosities of the vein is due to weakening of the valves and the walls of the vein

Thrombophlebitis is a condition where there is formation of a thrombus in vein with inflammatory changes

Discussions

- Name few medium-sized veins.
- Enumerate the layers of medium-sized vein with its constituents.
- Why do not you expect the vasa vasorum in the adventitial layer of medium-sized vein?
- What is a valve? What is its function?
- List the histological differences between medium-sized artery and medium-sized vein.
- What is thrombophlebitis?

CHAPTER

12 Integumentary System

INTRODUCTION

- Skin and its appendages are collectively put together in integumentary system (Fig. 12.1).
- Skin is of two types, i.e. thick skin and thin skin (Table 12.1). Skin appendages include sweat gland, sebaceous gland, nail and hair.

SKIN

- Skin is the largest organ in the body, which forms about one sixth of the total body weight of an individual.
- There are two types of skin, i.e. thick skin and thin skin, and histologically skin has two layers—inner dermis and outer epidermis (Fig. 12.2).

THICK SKIN

Slide No. 24

Identification Points

- Thick epidermis of stratified squamous keratinized epithelium
- Prominent dermal and epidermal papillae
- Absence of hair follicles.

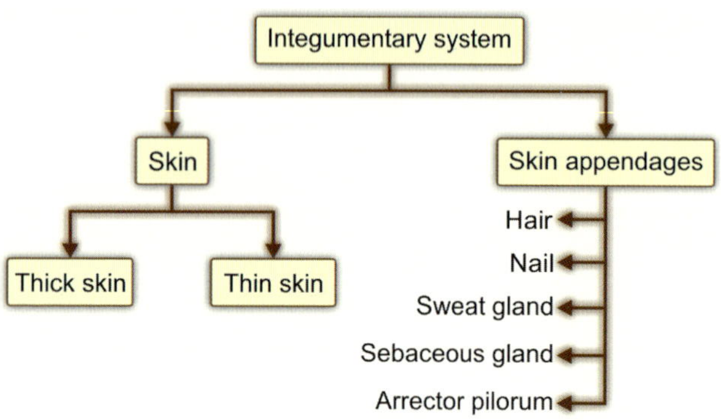

Figure 12.1: Integumentary system

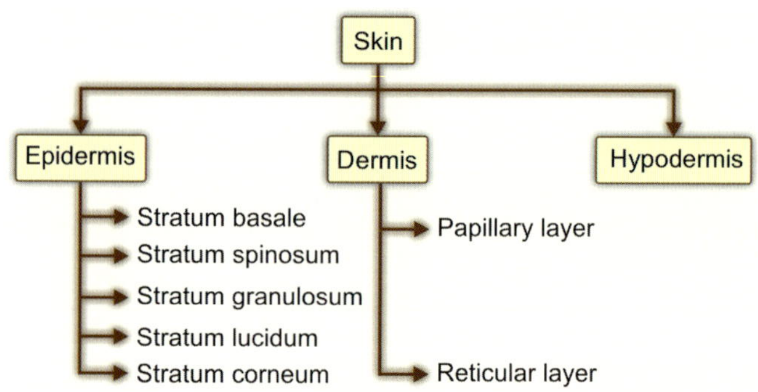

Figure 12.2: Layers of skin

Table 12.1: Difference between thick skin and thin skin

Thick skin	Thin skin
Epidermis layer is more thickened	Epidermis layer is less thickened
Corneal layer is very prominent	Corneal layer is very thin
Dermal papillae are better visualized	Dermal papillae are not so good to appreciate
Hair follicles are absent	Hair follicles are present
Location: Sole of the foot and palm of the hand	Location: All other parts of skin except the sole and palm
Sebaceous glands are absent	Sebaceous glands are present

Structure

Thick skin (Figs 12.3A and B) consists of outer epidermal layer and inner dermal layer, which can be explained below.

Epidermis: It is an outermost layer of thick skin consisting of following different layers of cells.

Stratum basale: It is the basal cell layer made up of simple columnar epithelium. Here all the cells are mitotically active and resting on basement membrane. Other than stem cells, it contains few melanocytes, Merkel cells and keratinocytes in it.

Stratum spinosum: Just above the basal layer there lies a multicellular layer made up of several polygonal cells:

- These cells are attached to each other by numerous desmosomes, which give a spine like appearance on the cells, hence the name **stratum spinosum.**
- This cell layer is also called **prickle cell layer** or **Malpighi cell layer** and few Langerhans. Cells are also seen in this layer.

Stratum granulosum: It is a thin layer of flattened cells found just above the stratum spinosum. Cell of this layer contains many basophilic keratohyalin granules in it. Hence, the name **stratum granulosum**.

Stratum lucidum: This is an amorphous clear, homogenized cell layer seen above the stratum granulosum. Here the cells are flat with no differentiating cell boundaries and, a flat nuclei here and there. This layer is well developed in thick skin.

Stratum corneum: It is the outermost layer of epidermis of thick skin seen beneath the stratum lucidum:

- Here all the cells are flat, dead with no nuclei and cell boundaries.
- This layer is rich in keratin, which acts as water proof to the skin.
- Prominent stratum corneum is seen in thick skin whereas it is very thin or absent in thin skin.

Dermis: This is the inner layer of thick skin seen below the epidermal layer. Dermis of the thick skin tries to invaginate

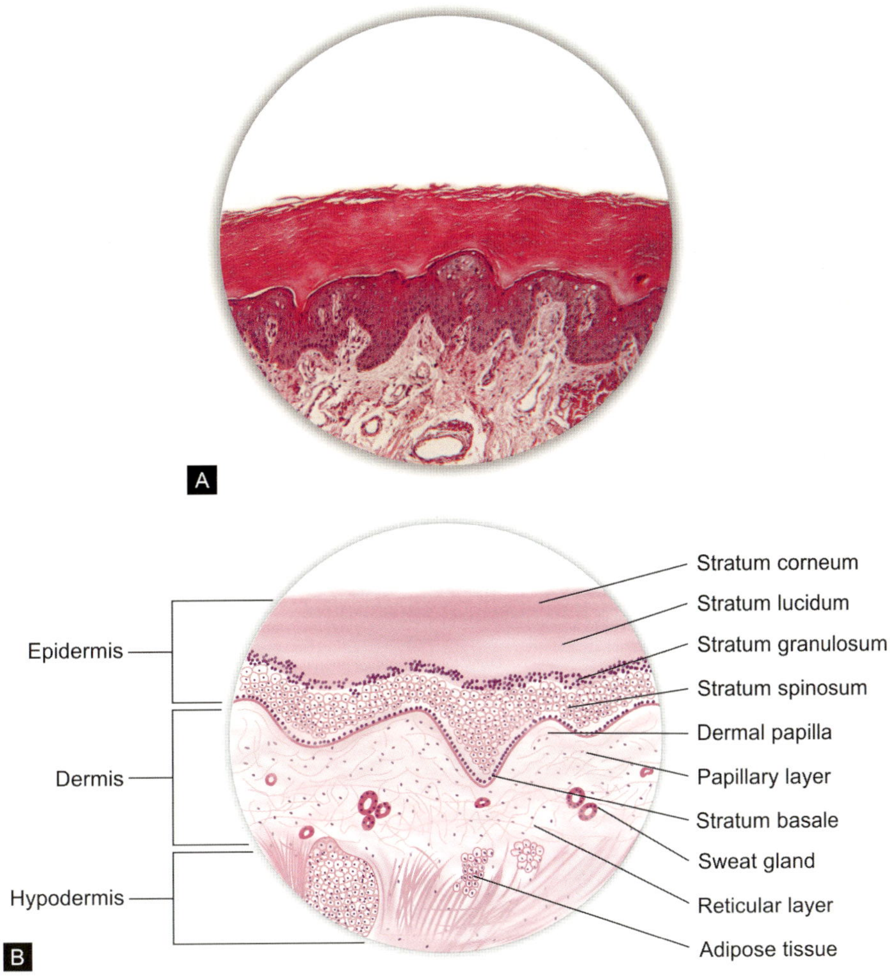

Figures 12.3A and B: Layers of thick skin. **A.** Photograph; **B.** Diagrammatic representation.

Clinical Histology
Psoriasis is a chronic inflammatory disease of the skin characterized by the formation of brownish red papules and plaques covered by silvery-white scales. It is due to the continuous stimulation of the stratum basale leading to increased mitotic cell division.
Squamous cell carcinoma is a skin cancer mainly arising from the cells of stratum spinosum.
Usually melanocytes are uniformly distributed in the skin, which gives a uniform color to the skin, but sometimes during the developmental stage a huge number of melanocytes aggregate in certain parts of the skin forming a **mole or nevi**.
Deficiency of melanin pigment results in white skin, if the white skin is in the form of few patches, it is known as **Leukoderma**. If it is uniform throughout, then it is referred as **Albinism.**
Hyperkeratosis is the term given to increased thickness of stratum corneum layer.

into the epidermis in the form of papillae known as **dermal papillae.** Similarly, downward projections of epidermis into the dermis form the **epidermal papillae (ridges)**.

Different layers of dermis are:

Papillary layer: It is an outer layer of dermis, rich in loose areolar connective tissue and blood capillaries in it. Dermal papillae containing **Meissner's corpuscles** are seen in this layer.

Reticular layer: It is an inner layer of dermis seen below the papillary layer. It chiefly consists of irregular bundles of collagen fibers with few elastic fibers in it. Appendages of the skin are usually present in this area along with few adipocytes and muscles in it.

Hypodermis: The layer below the dermis is called hypodermis. Hypodermis of the thick skin contains two sensory receptors called Pacinian corpuscles.

Apart from this, hypodermis is rich in adipose tissue and muscle fibers in it.

Discussions

- Name the layers of skin.
- Name the layers of epidermis. Which layer is also called as prickle cell layer?
- Name the layers of dermis. Which layer is rich in reticular fibers in it?
- Which is the outermost layer of epidermis? What does it contain?
- What are Meissner's corpuscles?
- What is keratin? What is its function?
- In which layer do you see melanocytes?
- What are dermal and epidermal papillae?
- What is hypodermis? What does it contain?
- What is albinism?

THIN SKIN

Slide No. 25

Identification Points

- Thin epidermis of stratified squamous non-keratinized epithelium
- Unmarked dermal and epidermal papillae
- Hair follicles with sebaceous glands and arrector pili muscles.

Structure

Thin skin consists of outer epidermis and inner dermal layer (Figs 12.4A and B).

Epidermis: Here the epidermis is thin with the presence of four layers, i.e. stratum basale, stratum spinosum, stratum corneum and stratum granulosum . Stratum lucidum is absent in thin skin.

Dermis: Dermis of the thin skin is same as that of thick skin in its composition except the smaller dermal papillae. In addition to this, dermis also contains hair follicles and arrector pili muscles attached to it. Numerous sebaceous glands are also present near the hair follicle to nourish it.

Clinical Histology
Infection of the sebaceous glands causes accumulation of sebum within the gland resulting into the formation of **sebaceous cyst** and is more common in scalp region
Infection of the hair follicle is called **folliculitis**

Discussions

- Name the layers of epidermis in thin skin.
- Which epidermal layers are absent in thin skin?
- Name the skin appendages present in dermis of thin skin.

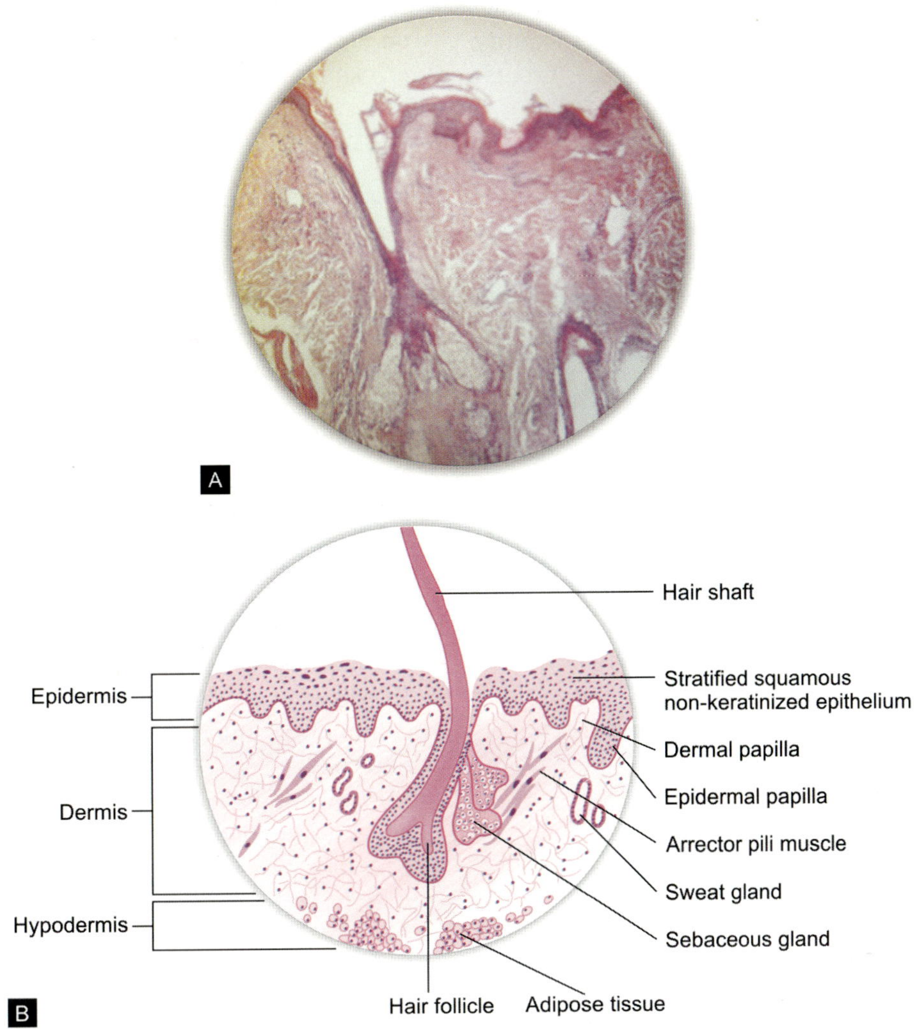

Figures 12.4A and B: Layers of thin skin. **A.** Photograph; **B.** Diagrammatic representation.

- What is the difference between dermal papillae of thick skin and thin skin?
- List the differences between thick skin and thin skin.
- Where do you see arrector pili muscles ?
- Enumerate the functions of skin.
- What is sebaceous cyst?
- What is folliculitis?

FUNCTIONS OF SKIN

- Acts as a mechanical barrier between the external environment and internal environment of body.
- Provides protection to the underlying tissues.
- Plays an important role in regulation of water and body temperature.
- Melanocytes present in the skin prevent cell injury caused by ultraviolet radiations of sun.
- Keratin, a sulfur containing protein of the skin is antibacterial in action and prevents skin infections.
- There are many receptors for heat, cold and temperature on the skin surface hence skin also acts as a sensory organ, etc.

SKIN APPENDAGES

Sweat Glands

Sweat glands are the simple tubular merocrine glands situated deep to the dermis or the upper hypodermis:

- A typical sweat gland is highly coiled structure with two different parts named secretory part and excretory (conductory) part.

- Secretory part consists of large columnar cells surrounded by few myoepithelial cells, whereas excretory part includes excretory duct, which traverses through dermis and opens into epidermis.

Functions

- Sweat gland produces sweat through which it maintains the body temperature and water balance.
- Unwanted toxic substances are excreted out of body through the sweat glands and its secretion.
- Sweat gland also plays an important role in electrolyte balance.

Sebaceous Glands

- Sebaceous glands (Fig. 12.5) are the holocrine glands found everywhere on skin except the palm and sole, and usually it is in association with the hair follicles.
- Sebaceous glands are made up of sebaceous cells containing a small round nuclei and an abundant fatty substance in it.
- The secretions of sebaceous gland is known as sebum.

Functions

- Sebaceous gland nourishes the hair follicle cells for its growth.
- Sebum from the gland acts as a protective covering on nipple, labia minora, prepuce and prevents it from cracking.

HAIR

Hair is present all over the body except palm, sole and some parts of male and female external genitalia:

- A typical hair (Fig. 12.6) has got a **shaft** present above the level of skin and a root underneath the skin.
- Lower pole of the root expands to form **bulb**, this bulb is invaginated by a part of dermis forming **hair papilla**.
- The root of each hair is surrounded by epithelial and connective tissue components forming, **hair follicle** and cut section of a hair shaft shows an outer cuticle layer, intermediate cortex and inner medulla.

NAIL

Nail is the thickening of the deep part of the stratum corneum of the skin:

- The distal part of nail is free whereas its proximal part is implanted into a groove on the skin and is called **nail root**.
- The **body** of the nail rests on **germinative zone,** which is richly supplied by the blood vessels that is why the nails look pink in color.

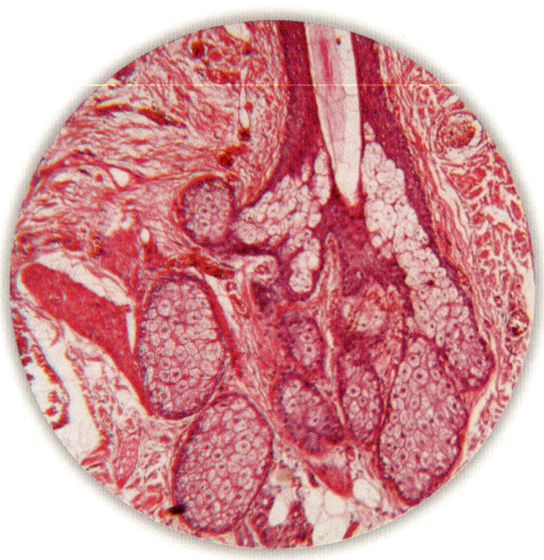

Figure 12.5: Sebaceous glands

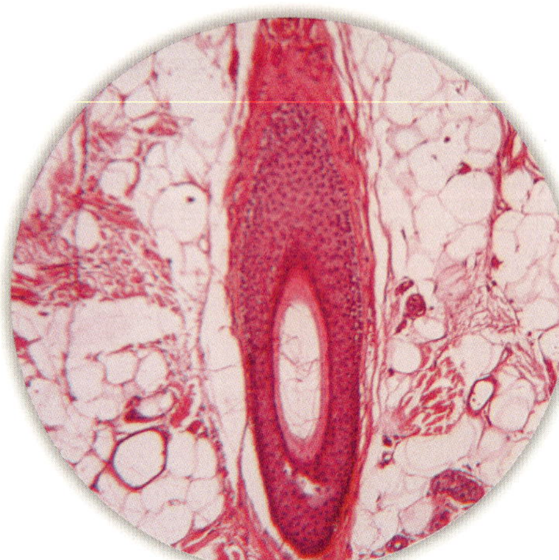

Figure 12.6: Hair follicles

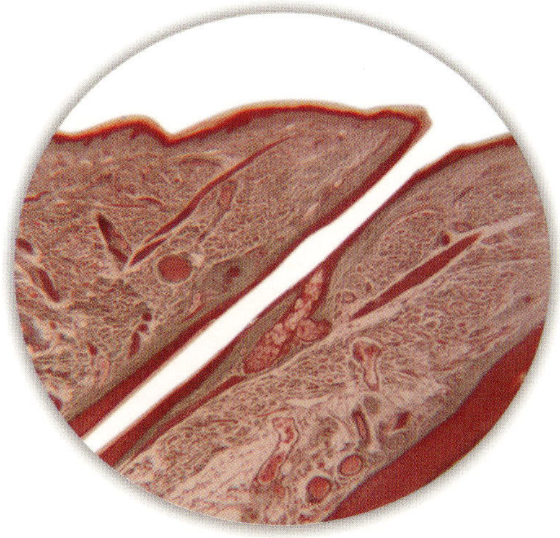

Figure 12.7: Arrector pilorum

ARRECTOR PILORUM

Arrector pilorum (Fig. 12.7) are the small bundles of smooth muscle fibers seen always in association with the hair follicle.

When these muscles contract, the hair become more erect and such a type of skin is known as **goose skin**.

SECTION 3

Systemic Histology

CHAPTER

13

Digestive System (Tooth and Tongue)

TOOTH (LS)

Slide No. 26

Identification Points

- Outermost enamel
- Prominent dentin with dentinal tubules
- Dental pulp containing blood vessels and nerve fibers in it.

Introduction

- Tooth is an accessory structure in the digestive system, which aids the process of mastication.
- Basically there are four types of teeth, i.e. incisors, canines, premolars and molars. All the teeth are placed in a bony, sac-like structure called **alveoli**.
- Human teeth are said to be **thecodont**, **diphyodont** and **heterodont**.

Structure

A longitudinal section of a tooth shows three majors parts (Fig. 13.1):

- **Crown:** It is the exposed and visible part of the tooth seen above the level of gingival epithelium.
- **Root:** It is the inner and deeper part of the tooth, which is placed in a bony socket called alveolus.
- **Neck:** It is a small constricted area, which connects the crown and the root. A detailed structure of the tooth can be explained as follows.

Enamel: It is a tough, rigid structure found in covering the crown of the dentin:

- Enamel is said to be the hardest structure in the body.
- It is made up of 96%–98% inorganic materials, 2%–4% organic materials.
- Organic material includes proteins **enamelin** and **amelogenin**, whereas hydroxyapatite crystals rich in calcium phosphate salts forms the inorganic part of it.

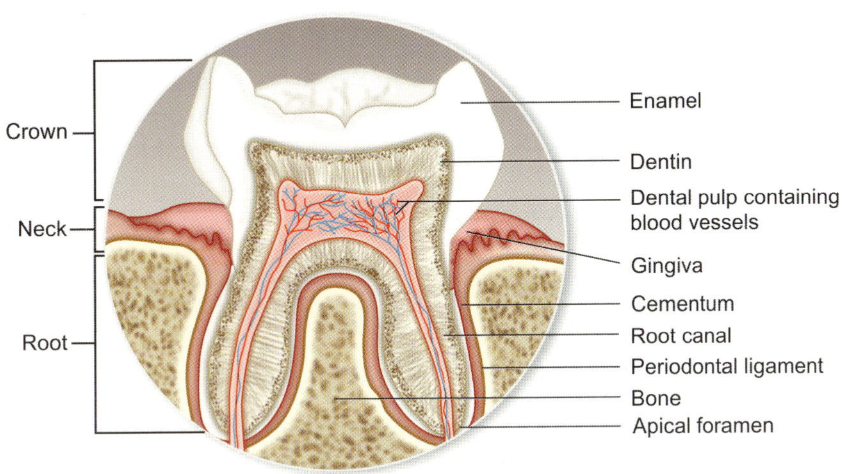

Figure 13.1: Tooth [longitudinal section (LS)]

- A layer of columnar cells present in an unerupted tooth called **ameloblasts** are known to produce the enamel and these ameloblasts degenerate permanently during of eruption of teeth.
- Enamel consists of numerous rods extending from dentin enamel junction to its free surface in the form of many layers. In between the two layers there is a brown line, which appears as an arching line and is called **Lines of Retzius**.

Dentin: It is a sensitive structure, which forms the main bulk of the tooth:

- The crown of the dentin is covered by enamel, whereas its lateral surfaces and root is protected by a layer of cementum.
- Dentin has a cavity at its center called **pulp cavity**. The wall of pulp cavity contains numerous **odontoblast** cells, which produce the dentin and their processes occupy dentinal tubules.

Pulp cavity: It is a cavity seen at the center of dentin, on either side it continues as **central canal or root canal**, which opens into the bony surface through an apical foramen:

- Pulp cavity is rich in pulp, i.e. loose areolar connective tissue through which numerous blood vessels and nerve fibers travel and anastomose with each other.
- These blood vessels and nerves leave the pulp cavity through apical foramen.

Cementum: It is a bony structure, which covers the root of dentin. It is produced by a modified osteoblast called **cementoblast**. Later they become cementocytes.

There are four types of cementum:

- Acellular.
- Cellular.
- Afibrillar.
- Intermediate.

Periodontal ligament: It is a layer of dense irregular connective tissue found in between the alveolar sockets and cementum:

- It is rich in densely packed collagen fibers collectively called **principal fibers**.
- The terminal ends of these fibers are deeply inserted into the substance of cementum and alveolar sockets, where they are called **Sharpey's fiber**.
- The periodontal ligament fixes the root of the tooth into the alveolar sockets firmly.

Gingiva (gum): It is a part of oral mucosa found in covering the neck of the tooth. It is composed of stratified squamous non-keratinized epithelium with a little amount of subendothelial connective tissue beneath it.

Clinical Histology
Progressive decay and disintegration of soft or bony tissue of tooth is termed as **Dental caries**. In this, dental enamel is destroyed exposing the dentin part, which is very sensitive to heat, cold and temperature. Hence, people with dental caries cannot drink hot tea and cold juices because of its intense pain and sensitivity.
Inflammation of alveolar socket of the tooth is known as **dentoalveolitis**. In severe condition it may lead to abscess formation.
Inflammation of the periodontal ligament is known as **periodontitis**.
Inflammation of the gums or gingiva is called **gingivitis**. It is characterized by redness, edema, bleeding tendencies and it is more common in tobacco chewers and people with bad oral hygiene.

Functions

- Tooth helps in mastication of the food particles.
- It aids the speech.
- To some extent it also counts in increasing face beauty.

Discussions

- What is a tooth? Name its different parts.
- Which is the hardest structure in the body?
- What is dentin?
- What is cementum and what is its function?
- What are odontoblasts? What do they do?
- List the different types of cementum.
- Where do you see the periodontal ligament?
- What are Sharpey's fibers?
- Which epithelium forms the gingiva or gums?
- What are dental caries?
- What is periodontitis?

TONGUE

CIRCUMVALLATE PAPILLA

Slide No. 27

Identification Points

- Lined by stratified squamous non-keratinized epithelium
- Numerous taste buds in the groove
- Presence of serous glands of von Ebner.

FILIFORM PAPILLA

Slide No. 28

Identification Points

- Finger-shaped structure
- Lined by stratified squamous keratinized epithelium
- Skeletal muscle protruding its substance.

FUNGIFORM PAPILLA

Slide No. 29

Identification Points

- Mushroom-shaped structure
- Lined by stratified squamous non-keratinized epithelium
- Skeletal muscle protruding its substance.

Introduction

- Tongue is a muscular organ lying on the floor of the oral cavity. In fact, it is the only skeletal muscle without the bony attachments. Let us know about its anatomy to understand its histology more better.
- Tongue has two surfaces with an apex and a base.
- Apex of the tongue points out whereas base is broad, fixed posteriorly.
- Dorsal surface of the tongue is divided into anterior two third and posterior one third by an inverted V- shaped groove called **sulcus terminalis**. The apex of V points backwards and is marked by a depression called **foramen cecum**.

Functions

Tongue helps in:

- Detection of taste
- Aids deglutition
- Helps in speech, etc.

Structure

Papilla

Since tongue is a muscular organ, most part of it is made up of skeletal muscles, which run in horizontal, vertical and longitudinal direction with the support of loose areolar connective tissue, whereas dorsal surface of the tongue is covered by mucous membrane lined by stratified squamous non-keratinized epithelium. Apart from this, mucous membrane of the tongue also bears numerous projections on its dorsal surface and are called **papillae**.

The various types of papillae are as given below.

a. **Circumvallate papilla (Figs 13.2A and B):**
   - These are the largest papillae of the tongue seen in front of the sulcus terminalis and they are 8–12 in number.
   - These papillae are having broad circular top with narrow base separated from rest of the part by a groove or a trench on the side called **vellum**. Hence, the name circumvallate papillae.

   Structure: It is lined by stratified squamous non-keratinized epithelium with a thick layer of connective tissue underneath it. Base of the papillae contains many circular and longitudinal muscle fibers projecting into its substance:

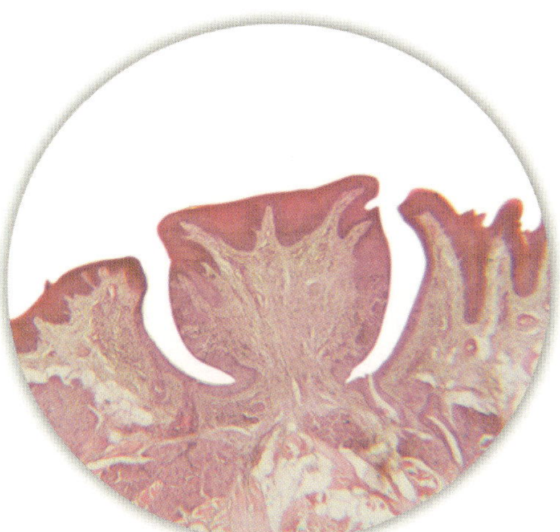

A

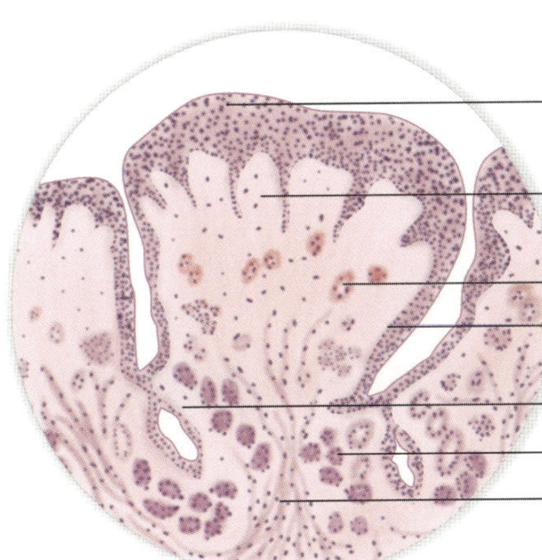

B

Figures 13.2A and B: Circumvallate papilla. **A.** Photograph; **B.** Diagrammatic representation.

- There are numerous serous glands seen near the base and groove of the papillae called **serous glands of von Ebner**.
- Its serous secretion helps in appreciating the taste of the food by dissolving the food particles in it.
- Groove of the papilla contains many taste buds in it with the opening of ducts of serous glands.

b. **Filiform papilla (Figs 13.3A and B):**

- These are numerous in number and situated widely on the dorsal surface of the tongue with a uniform distribution.
- Filiform papilla is a finger-like structure with a slender conical projection on it and is lined by stratified squamous non-keratinized epithelium with a partial keratinization at its tip. Few glands and muscles fibers may be seen near its base with few or no taste buds.

c. **Fungiform papilla (Figs 13.4A and B):**

- Fungiform papillae are seen at the apex of the tongue along with the lateral sides of the tongue.
- It is a large papilla with a lining of stratified squamous non-keratinized epithelium on its surface.
- A fungiform papilla is large blunt elevation with rounded summits having a short base with few taste buds on its groove and surface.
- Along with muscle fibers few serous glands are also seen near its base, which open into its groove.

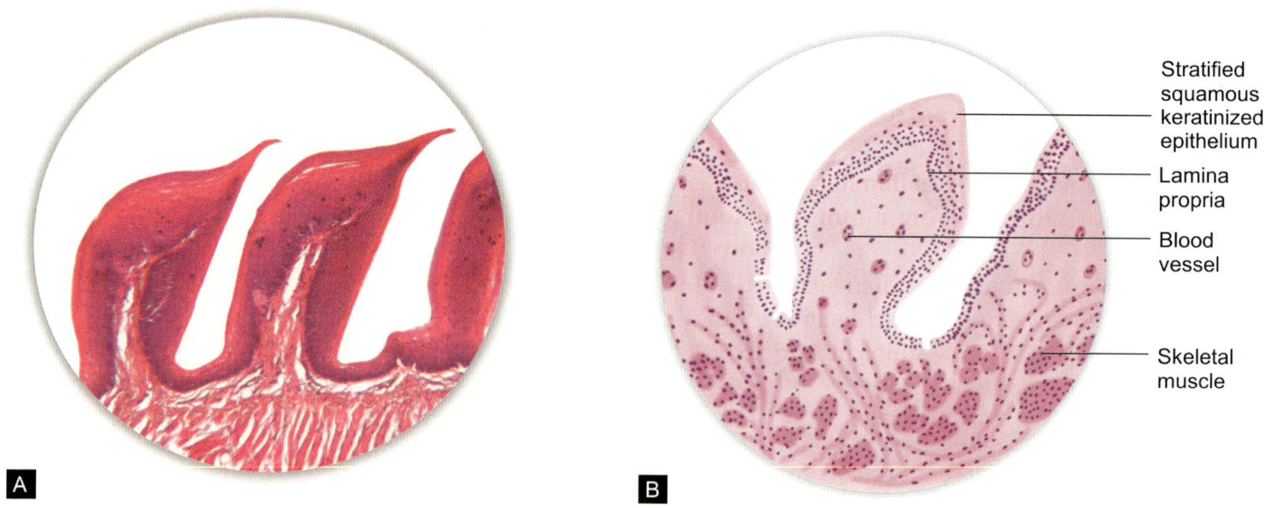

Figures 13.3A and B: Filiform papilla. **A.** Photograph; **B.** Diagrammatic representation.

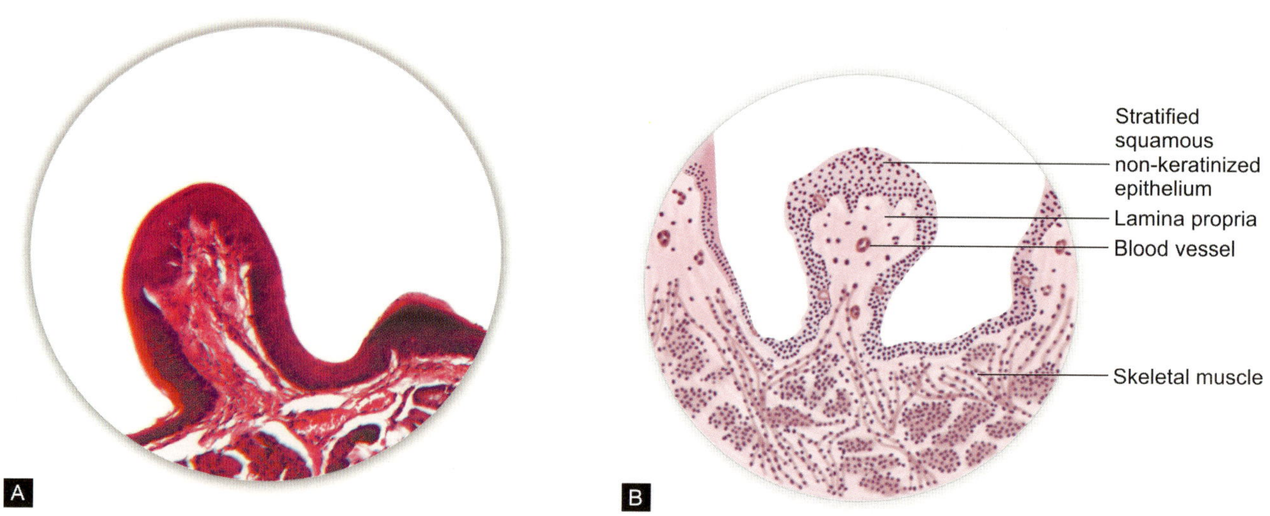

Figures 13.4A and B: Fungiform papilla. **A.** Photograph; **B.** Diagrammatic representation.

d. **Foliate papillae:**
   - These are the papillae with a shape of leaf found to be rudimentary in men, but functional in lower animals such as cows and buffaloes.

Taste buds

- Taste buds (Fig. 13.5) are the active centers of taste appreciation located on the different papillae of the tongue.
- Taste buds are numerous in circumvallate papillae and are located near its groove, whereas they are very few or almost absent in case of filiform papillae. Fungiform papillae bear the taste buds either on its surface or in its groove or both; but they are relatively less than that of taste buds in circumvallate papillae.
- A typical taste bud is a barrel or piriform-shaped structure made up of modified epithelial cells.
- Taste buds are made up of three different types of cells with a gustatory pores at its apex and the cells are the following.

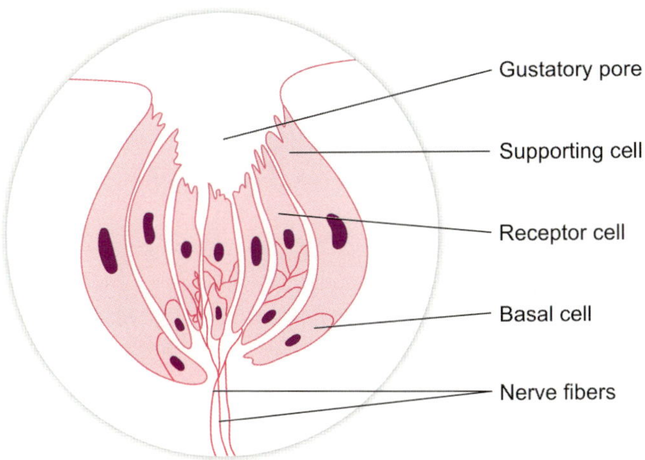

Figure 13.5: Taste bud

Gustatory cells or receptor cells: These are the bipolar neuroepithelial cells with lightly stained cytoplasm. Upper pole of this cell bears fine microvilli whereas the lower pole is in association with sensory nerve fibers.

Supportive or sustentacular cells: These are long elongated epithelial cells with a darkly stained nucleus and cytoplasm. They also bear fine microvilli at its upper pole and the lower pole is close to the basal cells.

Basal cells or stem cells: These are small pyramidal cells lying close to the basement membrane of the epithelium.

Functions

- Receptor cells are specialized for perception of the taste.
- Supportive cells aid the function of receptor cells and is supportive in function.
- Basal cells are the active stem cells, which give rise to receptor cells and supportive cells.

Clinical Histology
Inflammation of the tongue is called **glossitis**.
Even though there are no specific taste buds for specific tastes, but few parts of the tongue perceive some tastes more better than the other part of the tongue. For example, sour is best appreciated over dorsum of tongue whereas sweet is appreciated better at the tip, salt by the area just behind the tip and bitter by circumvallate papillae and posterior part of the tongue. Usually liquid foods are better appreciated by the taste buds than the solid foods.
Posterior one third of the tongue is rich in small lymphoid aggregations, which are collectively called **lingual tonsils** and they also contain many mucous glands.

Discussions

- What is sulcus terminalis?
- What is foramen cecum? What is its importance?
- Name the different muscles of the tongue.
- List the different papillae of the tongue with its location.
- What are serous glands of von Ebner? What is its function?
- Which papilla is rudimentary in human beings?
- Name the papilla with a partial keratinization over its surface.
- What are gustatory pores?
- What is a taste bud? Name the different cells of taste buds with its function.
- Which part of the tongue is rich in lingual tonsils?

CHAPTER 14

Digestive System (Salivary Glands)

SALIVARY GLANDS

Salivary glands are one of the important accessory organs of digestive system, which helps in better digestion and absorption of food. Following are the types of classification of salivary glands.

Classification I (Based on the Size and Amount of Saliva Secretion)

- Major salivary glands: There are three pairs of major salivary glands, which contribute about 90% of the total salivary secretion and they are parotid salivary gland, submandibular salivary gland and sublingual salivary gland.
- Minor salivary glands: There are many unpaired small salivary glands in the oral cavity, which contribute about 10% of the total salivary secretion and they are buccal gland, labial gland and palatal gland.

Classification II (Based on the Type of Secretion) (Figs 14.1A to C)

- Serous salivary gland: It is a type of salivary gland, which is predominantly made up of serous glands and they secrete thin watery saliva, e.g. parotid salivary gland.

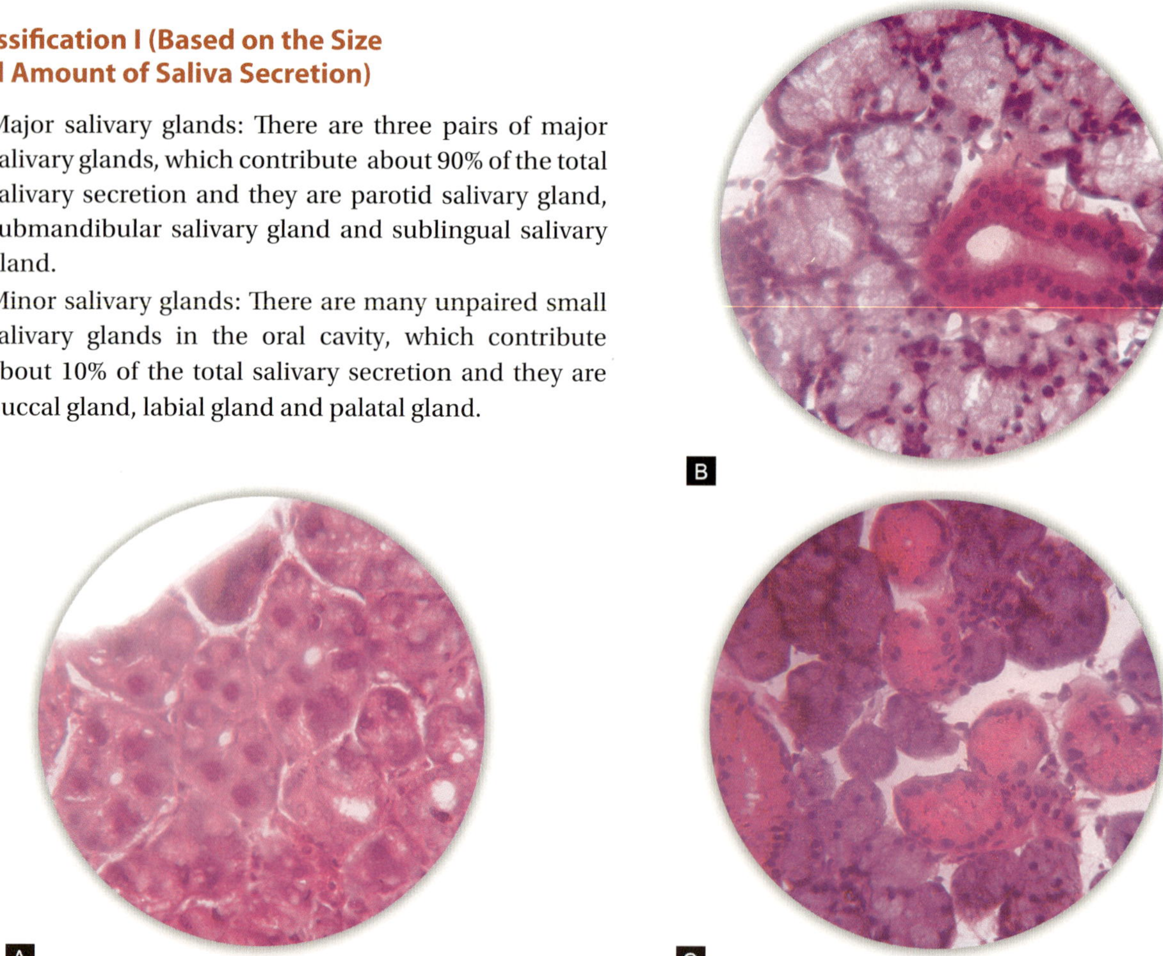

Figures 14.1A to C: Salivary glands. **A.** Serous; **B.** Mucous; **C.** Mixed type (Note the cellular differences between these types).

- Mucous salivary gland: It is a type of salivary gland, which is predominantly made up of mucous glands and they secrete thick mucinous saliva, e.g. sublingual salivary gland.
- Mixed salivary gland: It is a type of salivary gland, which is made up of both serous and mucous salivary glands, e.g. submandibular salivary gland.

PAROTID SALIVARY GLAND

Slide No. 30

Identification Points

- Serous acini with narrow lumen (Figs 14.2A and B)
- Centrally placed round nuclei
- Numerous ducts are present.

Introduction

- Parotid gland is a major salivary gland situated in front and slightly below the ear.
- The secretions of the gland are serous in nature. Hence, the gland is also known as **serous salivary gland.**
- It is said to be a **compound tubuloalveolar gland (racemose gland).**

Structure

A detailed structure of the parotid salivary gland can be explained as follows.

Capsule: It is an outermost part of the gland made up of dense irregular connective tissue and the deep cervical fascia splits up into two layers to enclose the parotid gland, which forms a pseudocapsule of the gland. The capsule of the gland sends many septae, which splits the parenchyma into many lobes and lobules.

Parenchyma: It is in the form of many lobes and lobules. A lobule is made up of many serous acini and a serous acini is lined by pyramidal shaped serous cells resting on basement membrane with a small lumen at the center.

Serous cell: A serous cell is a modified epithelial cell with a broad base and tapering apex pointing toward the lumen. Here, the cell surface bears numerous microvilli on it:

- Each serous cell has a round nucleus at the center with numerous zymogen granules at its tip and an abundant rough endoplasmic reticulum at its base. Thus the apex is brightly stained with pink color, whereas base takes purple color because of its staining property.
- Thus the serous acinar cells are **biphasic** in nature.
- In between the acini, there is stroma made up of loose areolar connective tissue with numerous ducts of varying size and few epitheliocytes surrounding the acini.

Duct system: There is an extensive variety of ducts system seen in the parotid gland, which is a special feature of it.

Following are the different types of ducts seen in the histology of parotid salivary gland:

- **Intercalated ducts:** These are the minute ducts lined by simple cuboidal epithelium. Here serous cells pour their secretions into lumen and the secretion is drained by these intercalated ducts.
- **Striated ducts:** These are slightly bigger than intercalated ducts and are lined by simple columnar epithelium containing many striations at its base; hence they are called striated ducts. These are located within the

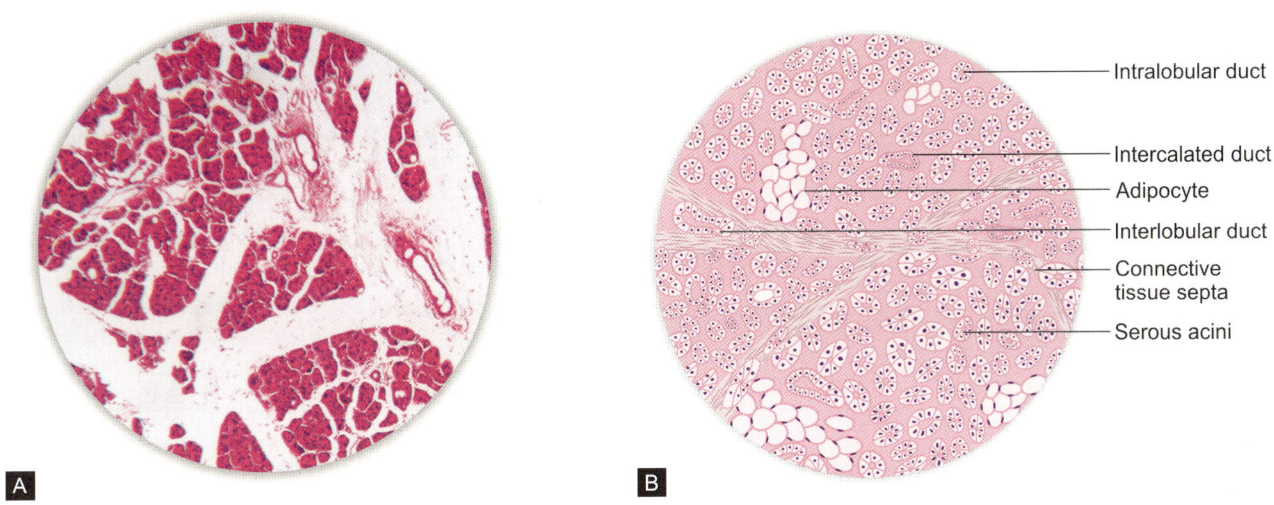

Figures 14.2A and B: Parotid salivary gland. **A.** Photograph; **B.** Diagrammatic representation.

lobules of the gland and drain the saliva or secretions from intercalated ducts.

- **Intralobular ducts:** These are slightly bigger than the striated ducts and are lined by simple columnar epithelium. These ducts are situated within the lobules and drain the secretions from striated ducts.
- **Interlobular ducts:** These are formed by the union of many intralobular ducts and are lined by pseudostratified columnar epithelium layer and these ducts drain the secretion from intralobular duct.
- **Interlobar ducts:** It is formed by the union of many interlobular ducts and they open into excretory (lobar) duct.
- **Excretory ducts:** It is the major duct also called **Stensen's duct** and is lined by stratified columnar epithelium. It is formed by the union of many interlobar ducts, which finally opens opposite to the crown of the upper second premolar tooth.

Functions

An important function of parotid gland is to secrete watery saliva, which helps in:

- Mastication
- Speech
- Oral hygiene
- Digestion.

Clinical Histology
Salivary corpuscles are the lymphocytes present in saliva, which are due to the accidental escape of few lymphocytes from tonsillar area to the saliva.
Inflammation of the parotid gland is known as **parotitis.** It is characterized by swelling and severe pain the gland after the intake of food.
Formation of small stones in the Stensen's duct leads to the obstruction in the passage of saliva and the condition is called **sialolithiasis.**

Discussions

- Where is parotid gland located? Which type of gland is it?
- What is a serous acinus?
- Where do you see zymogen granules in the serous cells?
- Why is serous acinar cell said to be biphasic in nature?
- What are myoepithelial cells? Where do you see it? What is its function?
- List the different ducts present in the serous salivary gland with its inner epithelial lining.
- What is the another name for parotid duct?
- List the functions of saliva.
- What are salivary corpuscles?

SUBLINGUAL SALIVARY GLAND

Slide No. 31

Identification Points

- Mucous acini with a large lumen
- Flat nucleus placed near the base of the cell
- Very few ducts are present.

Introduction

- Sublingual salivary gland (Figs 14.3A and B) is one of the important salivary glands located just below the tongue; hence the name **sublingual salivary gland.**
- The secretion of the gland is predominantly mucous, hence also called **mucous salivary gland.**

Structure

A detailed structure of it can be explained under following headings.

Capsule: It is the outermost part of the gland made up of dense irregular connective tissue.

The capsule of the gland sends many septae, which splits the parenchyma into many lobes and lobules.

Parenchyma: Parenchyma of the gland is in the form of many lobes and lobules. A lobule is made up of many mucous acini:

- A mucous acini is lined by a truncated columnar epithelium resting on the basement membrane.
- Here, a mucous acinus is larger than the serous acinus with a large lumen at its center.

Mucous cell: A mucous cell is a large truncated columnar cell with a broad base and blunt apex pointing toward the lumen:

- Here the cell surface does not bear microvilli on it.
- Each mucous cell has a flat nucleus at its base and there are many secretory vesicles containing mucin in it.
- In between the acini, there is a stroma made up of loose areolar connective tissue and few epitheliocytes surrounding the acini.

Duct system: Duct system in sublingual salivary gland is same as that of parotid salivary gland, but its development is very poor here.

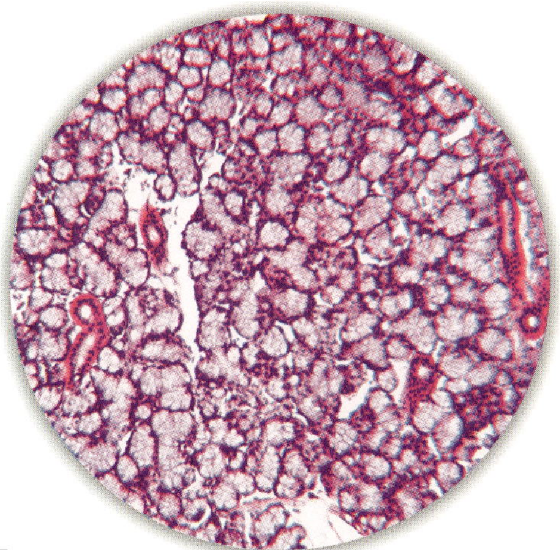

A

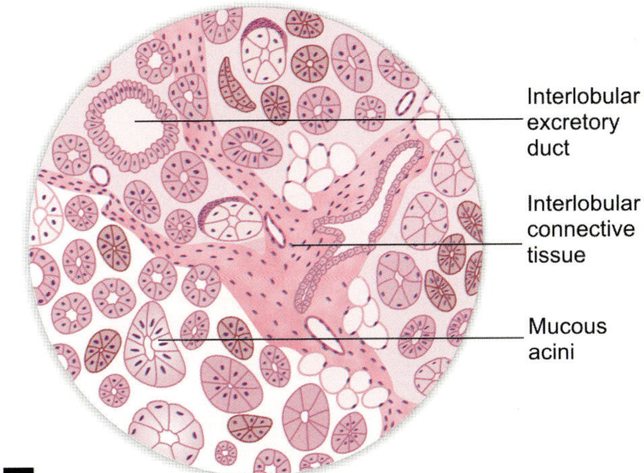

B

Figures 14.3A and B: Sublingual salivary gland. **A.** Photograph; **B.** Diagrammatic representation.

Functions

Like parotid gland, sublingual salivary gland also secretes saliva, which is thick mucus (Table 14.1) in nature and saliva does many functions, as described in previous discussions.

Discussions

- Where is sublingual salivary gland located?
- What is the another name for sublingual salivary gland? Why is it called so?
- What is a mucous acinus?
- List the differences between serous and mucous acinus.

Table 14.1: Differences between serous and mucous acini

Serous acinus	Mucous acinus
Small in size	Large in size
Lined by pyramidal shaped cells	Lined by truncated columnar cells
Has small, narrow lumen	Has large, broad lumen
Nucleus is round, placed at the center of cell	Nucleus is flat, placed toward the base of cell
Biphasic in nature	Not biphasic in nature
Apex of the cell contains zymogen granules	Apex of the cell contains mucigen droplets
Darkly stained	Lightly stained
Secretes thin watery saliva, e.g. parotid salivary gland	Secretes thick viscous saliva, e.g. sublingual salivary gland

SUBMANDIBULAR SALIVARY GLAND

Slide No. 32

Identification Points

- Both serous and mucous acini are seen
- Serous demilunes of Giannuzzi are present
- Few ducts are present.

Introduction

Submandibular salivary gland (Figs 14.4A and B) is located below the body of the mandible; hence it gets its name as **submandibular salivary gland.**

Structure

Histologically, it is made up of both serous and mucous acini; thus, it is also named as **mixed salivary gland.** But it is predominatly serous type in nature. It can be explained as follows.

Capsule: It is the outermost protective covering of the gland made up of dense irregular connective tissue, which sends many septae into the gland, thus dividing the gland into various lobes and lobules.

Lobules: Even though the lobules of the gland are made up of both serous and mucous acini, serous cells predominate over mucous cells and serous cells form a crescent or moon-shaped cap over the mucous cells known as **Crescent of Giannuzzi** or **Demilunes of Heidenhain.**

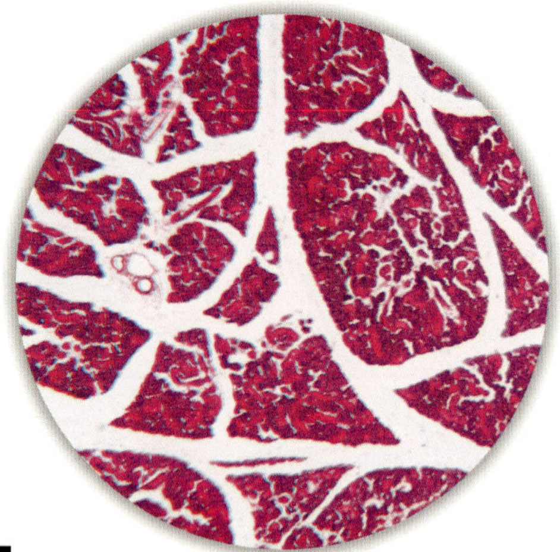

A

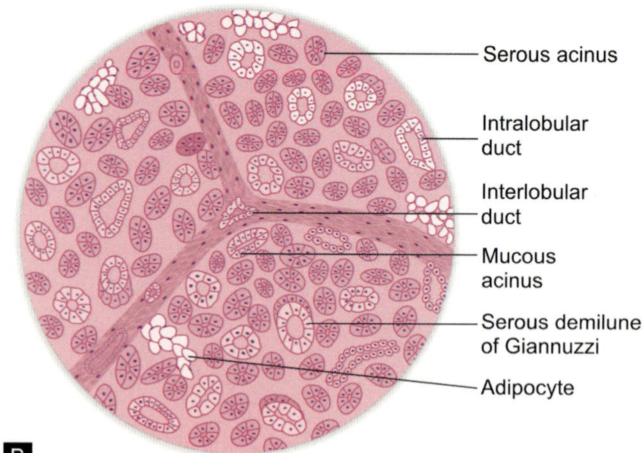

B

Figures 14.4A and B: Submandibular salivary gland. **A.** Photograph; **B.** Diagrammatic representation.

Duct system: Duct system of submandibular salivary gland is same as that of parotid salivary gland, but its development is moderate when compared to parotid salivary gland.

Functions

Secretes saliva, which performs many functions, as mentioned in previous discussions.

Discussions

- Where is submandibular salivary gland located?
- What is the another name for submandibular salivary gland? Why is it called so?
- What are demilunes of Heidenhain?

CHAPTER

15 Digestive System (Esophagus and Stomach)

ESOPHAGUS (TS) (Figs 15.1A and B)

Slide No. 33

Identification Points

- Mucosa lined by stratified squamous non-keratinized epithelium
- Submucosa containing esophageal glands
- Muscularis externa containing inner circular and outer longitudinal muscle layer.

Introduction

- Esophagus is a hollow muscular tube-like structure, which extends from lower end of pharynx up to the cardiac end of stomach.
- On an average, length of esophagus is about 25 cm and is grossly divided into upper one third, middle one third and lower one third.
- Esophagus develops in 4th week of intrauterine life from **tracheoesophageal bud.**

Structure

A detailed structure of esophagus is explained under the following headings.

Mucosa: It is an innermost layer of esophagus lined by stratified squamous non-keratinized epithelium, which is resting on basement membrane. Here surface epithelium may contain few specialized cells belonging to APUD cell system (APUD stands for amine precursor uptake decarboxylase).

Lamina propria: Just beneath the epithelium there is a layer of loose connective tissue called **lamina propria** and is folded into many finger-like projections called papillae:

- Papillae help in firm attachment of surface epithelium to the underlying lamina propria

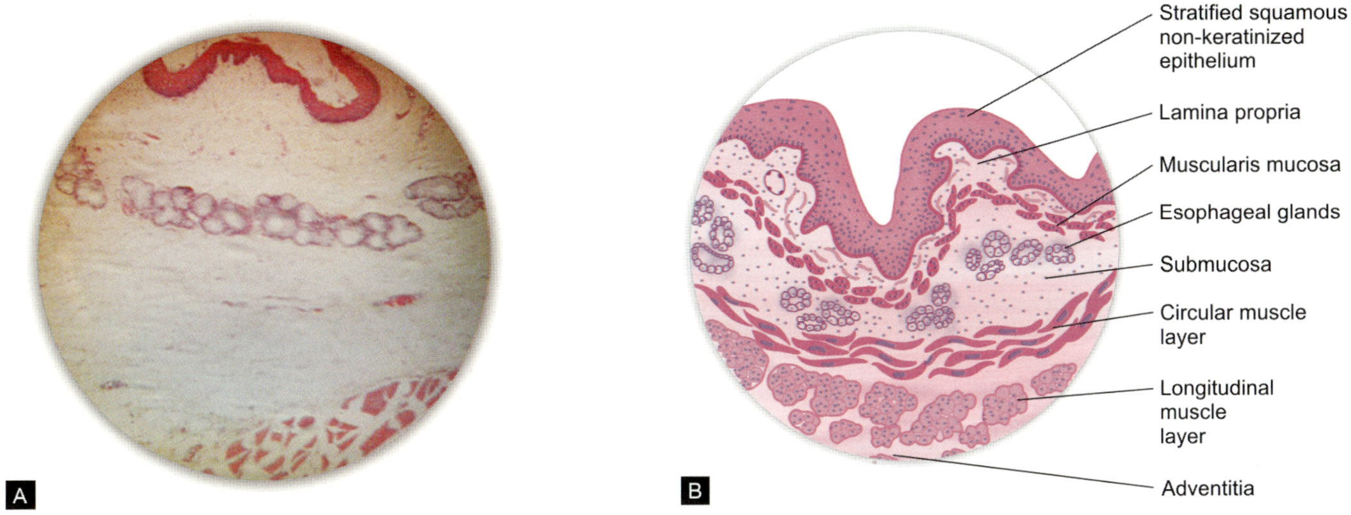

Figures 15.1A and B: Esophagus. **A.** Photograph; **B.** Diagrammatic representation.

- In lower one third of esophagus lamina propria may contain few small lymphoid aggregations and tubuloalveolar mucous glands.

Muscularis mucosa: It consists of a thin layer of bundles of longitudinal muscle fibers. It is said to be absent or poorly developed in upper one third of esophagus, moderately developed in middle one third and very distinct in lower one third of esophagus.

Submucosa: It is made up of loose areolar connective tissue rich in connective tissue fibers, cells and blood vessels. Submucosa of esophagus is characterized by the presence of numerous **compound tubulo-alveolar mucous glands** also called **esophageal glands.**

Muscularis externa: It is found just beneath the submucosa and consists of inner layer of circular muscles and outer layer of longitudinal muscle fibers:

- It is important to notice that in upper one third of esophagus, muscularis externa is said to be striated in nature, it is mixed with striated and smooth muscles in middle one third and is purely smooth muscle variety in lower one third of esophagus.
- It is assumed that the circular muscle fibers present in the lower end of esophagus may form cardioesophageal sphincter, but anatomically it is not accepted.

Adventitia: It is the outermost protective layer made up of dense irregular connective tissue.

Functions

- Surface epithelium lining the esophagus bares various mechanical and chemical injuries thus it protects the internal tissues from being damaged.
- Mucosal glands present in submucosa secretes mucus, which lubricates the surface epithelium thus protecting it against infections.
- Circular and longitudinal muscle fibers of muscularis externa contract powerfully thus propelling the food forwards by means of **peristalsis.**
- Adventitia is supportive and protective in function.

Clinical Histology
Reflux esophagitis is a clinical condition caused by the reflux of gastric juice from stomach to lower end of esophagus resulting in destruction of surface epithelium and inflammation
Due to repeated reflux esophagitis, stratified squamous non-keratinized epithelium of lower esophagus is replaced by columnar epithelium (columnar metaplasia) and the condition is known as **Barrett's esophagus**

Discussions

- Name the different layers of esophagus.
- Describe the mucosa of esophagus.
- Name the type of muscles seen in muscularis mucosa.
- What is the special feature of submucosa in esophagus?
- Name the muscular pattern seen in muscularis externa.
- What is an adventitia? What is it made up of?
- List the functions of different layers of esophagus.
- What is physiological sphincter?
- What is reflux esophagitis?

STOMACH (FUNDUS) (Figs 15.2A and B)

Slide No. 34

Identification Points

- Mucosa lined by simple columnar epithelium.
- Numerous chief and parietal cells in lamina propria.
- Muscularis externa containing inner oblique, middle circular and outer longitudinal muscle layer.

Introduction

- Stomach is a muscular bag-like structure, which stores the food temporarily for few hours
- It is divided into three major parts, i.e. fundus, body and pylorus.

A detailed structure of fundic part of stomach shows following features.

Mucosa

- Mucosa of fundic stomach is folded into many rugae, which disappear on expansion
- Mucosa is lined by simple columnar epithelia, which are resting on basement membrane
- Most of the places it dips into the underlying lamina propria forming walls of depression known as **gastric pits**
- Gastric pits are shallow in fundic part of stomach and form about one fourth of the total thickness of mucosa.

Lamina propria

Lamina propria of fundic part of stomach is rich in fundic glands consisting of following types of cells:

- **Stem cells:** These are the active, undifferentiated cells found at the base of lamina propria, which gives rise to all other types of cells.
- **Enteroendocrine cells:** These are the special type of cells found just above the stem cells. They are also called **argentaffin cells,** since they are stained by silver salts. They belong to **APUD cell system** and known to

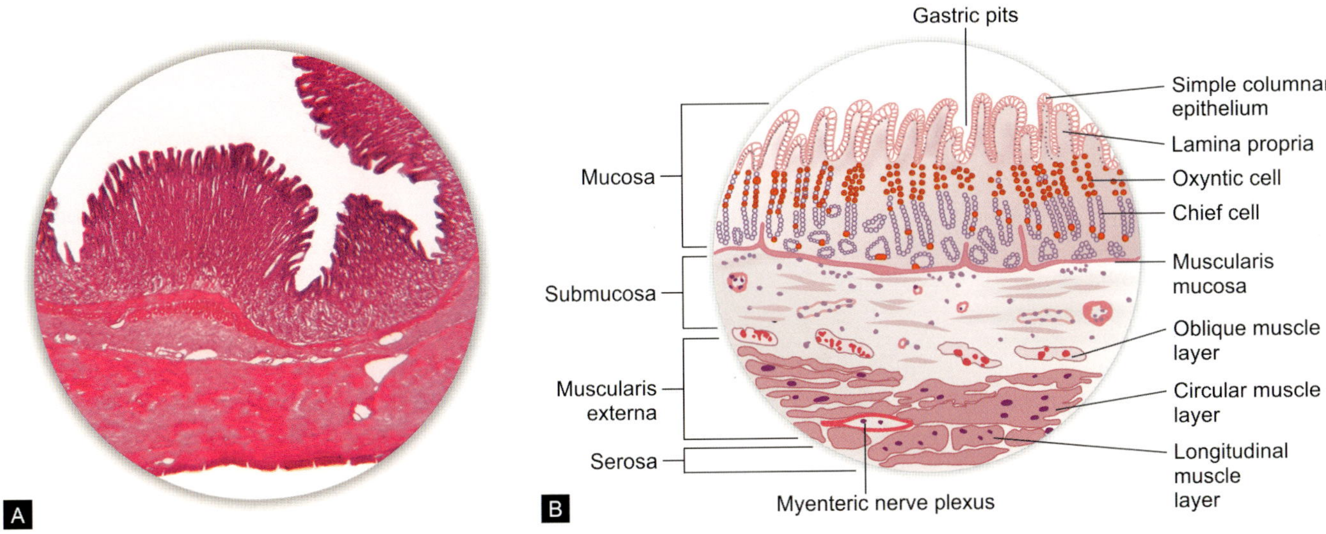

Figures15.2A and B: Stomach (fundus). **A.** Photograph; **B.** Diagrammatic representation.

produce some local hormones like **somatostatin** and **gastrin.**

- **Chief cells:** These are the small cuboidal cells, which lie upon the enteroendocrine cells:
  - They are very large in number with basophilic cytoplasm and few zymogen granules in them hence they are also referred to as **zymogenic cells**
  - As they produce protein digestive enzymes like pepsin (renin) some people also name them as **peptic cells.**
- **Oxyntic cells:** These are large pyramidal or polyhedral cells with central nucleus, found lying in between mucous neck cells and chief cells:
  - They are present in upper half of the lamina propria and are easily identified by its strong bright eosinophilic cytoplasm, hence it gets its name **oxyntic cells**
  - They are also called **parietal cells** as they lie against the basement membrane of surface epithelium giving beaded appearance.

    Their function is to secrete:
  - Hydrochloric acid, which is a part of gastric juice
  - Intrinsic factor, which is necessary for the absorption of vitamin B_{12} from gut system for erythropoiesis.
- **Mucous neck cells:** These are the low columnar cells present near neck of the gastric glands:
  - They are the large cells with flat nucleus at its base and whole cell is accumulated by acid mucus
  - They open into gastric pits and secrete acid mucus.

Muscularis mucosa

Muscularis mucosa consists of thin layer of inner circular and outer longitudinal muscle fibers extending into the lamina propria here and there.

Submucosa

- Submucosa is made up of loose areolar connective tissue, rich in connective tissue fibers and cells with many blood vessels in it
- It also contains **Meissner's plexus** of nerve fibers in it.

Muscularis externa

- Muscularis externa is made up of inner oblique, middle circular and outer longitudinal muscle layers
- In between circular and longitudinal muscle layer, few **myenteric (Auerbach's) plexus** of nerve fibers are seen.

Serosa

Serosa is an outermost layer made up of few connective tissue cells and fibers, covered by mesothelium of the visceral peritoneum.

Functions

- Simple columnar epithelium lining the mucosal surface has both secretory and absorptive functions, i.e. as a secretory part it secretes mucus and it also absorbs a small amount of alcohol and certain chemical drugs.
- Submucosa is defensive and nutritive in functions since it contains connective tissue cells and numerous blood vessels in it.

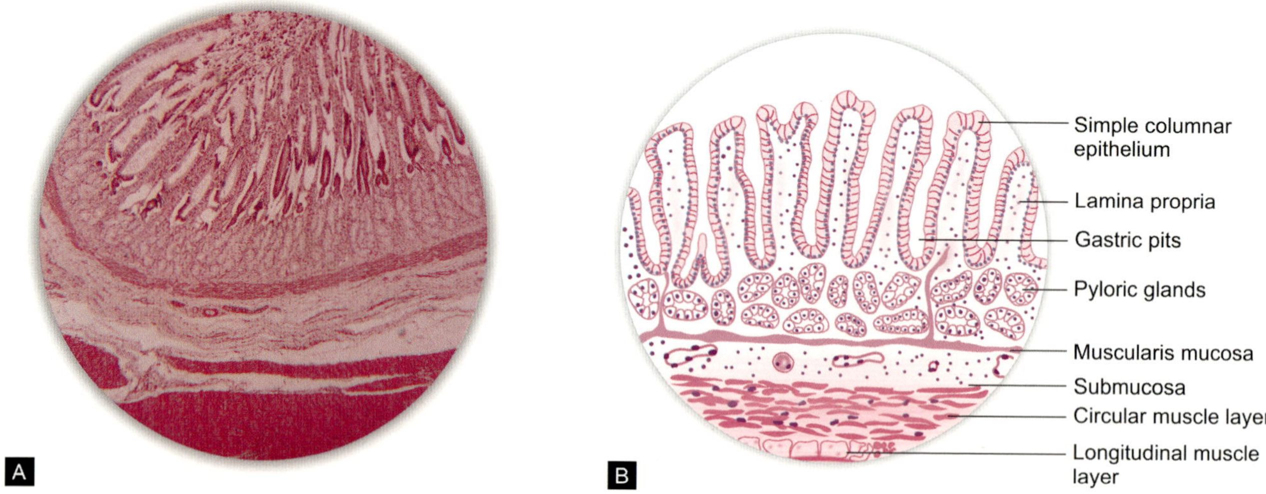

Figures 15.3A and B: Stomach (pylorus). **A.** Photograph; **B.** Diagrammatic representation.

- Muscularis externa containing different muscle layers help in churning the food particles and peristalsis by its powerful contractions.
- Serosa is supportive and protective in function.

Clinical Histology
Inflammation of gastric mucosa by *Helicobacter pylori* bacteria causes **gastritis**
Hypersecretion of acid HCl and pepsin enzymes from oxyntic cells and chief cells leads to degeneration and necrosis of gastric mucosa resulting in **peptic (gastric) ulcers**
Uncontrolled abnormal proliferation of surface epithelium of stomach leads to **gastric carcinoma**

Discussions

- Name the four layers of stomach.
- Which epithelium lines the mucosa of stomach?
- Name the different types of cells present in fundic glands of stomach with one function each.
- What are argentaffin cells? Why are they called so?
- Where do you see?
  - Meissner's plexus.
  - Myenteric plexus of nerve fibers.
- Describe the muscularis externa of stomach.
- Enumerate the functions of each layer of stomach.
- What is gastric ulcer?

STOMACH (PYLORUS) (Figs 15.3A and B)

Slide No. 35

Identification Points

- Deep gastric pits
- Lamina propria containing pyloric glands
- Thickened middle circular muscle layer forming pyloric sphincter.

Histology of pyloric part of stomach is almost same as that fundic part of stomach except few differences wherein pyloric part of stomach shows:

- Gastric pits forming about half of total thickness of gastric mucosa
- Lamina propria rich in mucous secreting **pyloric glands**
- Middle circular layer of muscularis externa becomes thicker than elsewhere forming **pyloric sphincter.**

Discussions

- What are the differences between pyloric part of stomach and fundic part of stomach?
- What are pyloric glands? What do they secrete?
- Which muscle layer is involved in formation of pyloric sphincter?

CHAPTER

16

Digestive System (Intestine and Pancreas)

INTRODUCTION

- Intestine of gastrointestinal system has got two parts—small intestine and large intestine.
- Small intestine consists of three parts, i.e. duodenum, jejunum and ileum. Large intestine consists of vermiform appendix, ascending colon, transverse colon, descending colon, sigmoid colon, rectum and anal canal (Fig. 16.1).

DUODENUM (TS)

Slide No. 36

Identification Points

- Numerous villi
- Crypts of Lieberkühn present
- Brunner's glands in submucosa.

Introduction

- Duodenum (Figs 16.2A and B) is the shortest segment of small intestine measuring about 25 cm.
- It is divided into four parts, i.e. superior part, descending part, horizontal part and ascending part.

Structure

A transverse section (TS) of duodenum shows following different layers.

Mucosa: It is the innermost layer of duodenum lined by simple columnar epithelium with fine microvilli at its tip. Few mucus secreting goblet cells are also present in surface epithelium:

- Here mucosa is thrown into minute finger like projections called **villi**. Villi help in increasing the surface area of absorption.

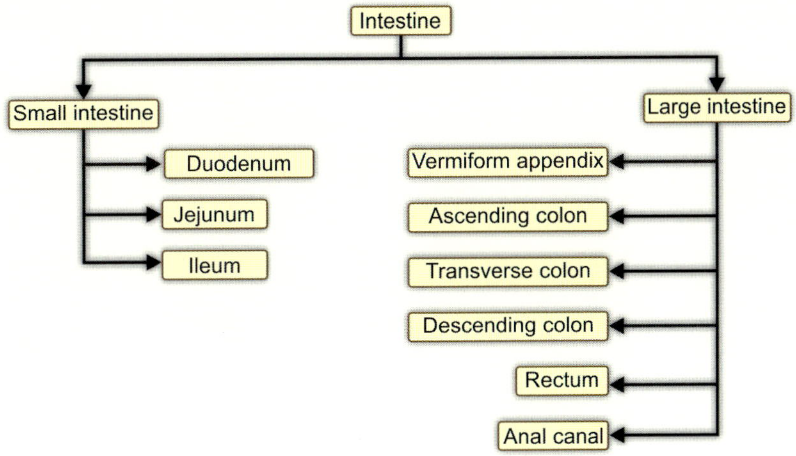

Figure 16.1: Classification of gastrointestinal system

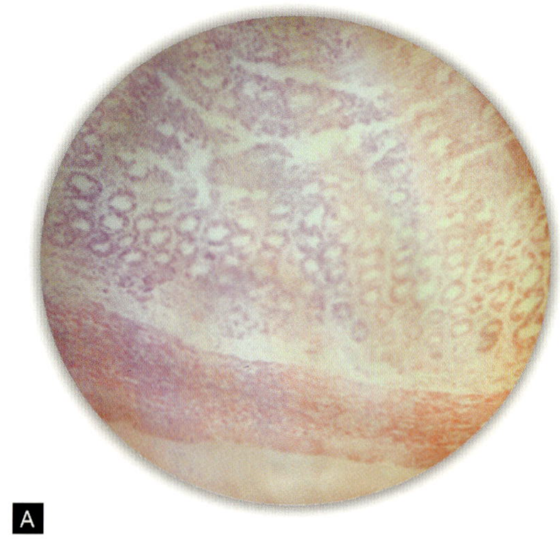

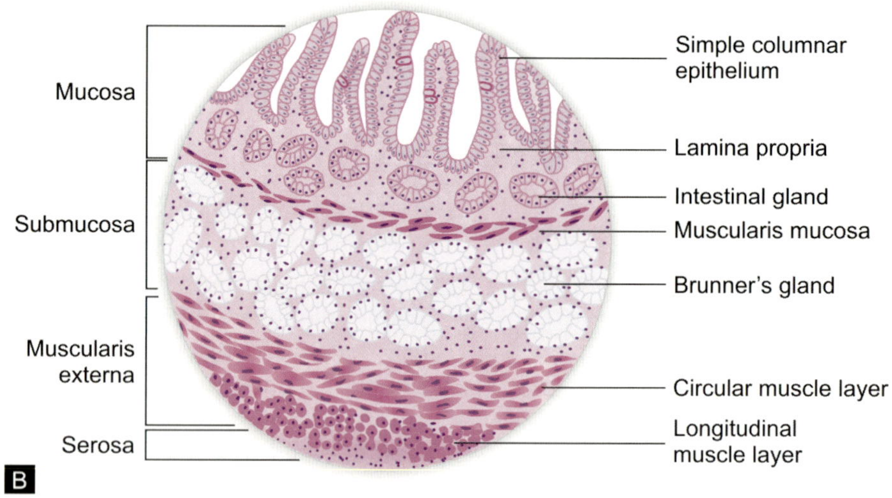

Figures 16.2A and B: Duodenum [transverse section (TS)]. **A.** Photograph; **B.** Diagrammatic representation.

- Typical villi is lined by surface epithelium and lamina propria projecting into it. It contains loose areolar connective tissue and a central core of lymphatics called **Lacteal**.
- Just below the mucosa their exists lamina propria containing simple tubular intestinal glands, which open into the crypts of villi and are also called **crypts of Lieberkühn**.

Crypts of Lieberkühn consist of following type of cells:

- *Stem cells:* These are the undifferentiated cells undergoing continuous mitotic cell division, which migrates, eventually replaces the old surface epithelium thus forming enterocytes.
- *Goblet cells:* They secrete mucus.
- *Enteroendocrine cells:* Also called **argentaffin cells**. They belong to APUD cell system and secrete local hormones such as secretin, cholecystokinin pancreozymin (APUD stands for amine precursor uptake and decarboxylation).
- *Paneth cells:* Also called **zymogenic cells** as they are rich in zinc and zymogen granules in it. They produce the digestive enzymes and lysosomes (antibacterial agents).

Muscularis mucosa: It is seen below the lamina propria and made up of thin layer of disrupted circular muscle fibers.

Submucosa: It contains loose areolar connective tissue with numerous mucus secreting duodenal glands called **Brunner's gland**:

- They secrete an alkaline fluid rich in bicarbonate.
- Combined secretion of Brunner's gland and intestinal glands is called **succus entericus.**

Muscularis externa: It is a muscular coat made up of inner circular and outer longitudinal muscle fibers in it.

- In between the two muscle layers few parasympathetic ganglionic cells of myenteric plexus can be seen.

Serosa: It is the outermost layer made up of connective tissue cells, adipocytes and few blood vessels. It is also blended by visceral peritoneum.

Functions

- Villi of duodenal mucosa are absorptive in function and they also increase the surface area of absorption.
- Brunner's glands present in submucosa secrete alkaline intestinal fluid helping in digestion.
- Muscularis externa propels the food forward by producing powerful contractions (peristalsis).
- Serosa is supportive and protective in function.

Discussions

- Name the surface epithelium lining the duodenal mucosa.
- What are villi? Describe its structure and function.
- What is lacteal?
- What are crypts of Lieberkühn and name its different component cells with one function each?
- What are Paneth cells? What do they produce?
- What is Brunner's gland? What do they secrete?
- Describe the following term:
  - Chyle.
  - Succus entericus.
- List the functions of different layers of duodenum.
- Enumerate the histological differences between stomach and duodenum.

JEJUNUM (TS)

Slide No. 37

Identification Points

- Tall villi lined by simple columnar epithelium with goblet cells
- Absence of Brunner's glands in submucosa
- Absence of Peyer's patches.

Structure

Histological features of jejunum (Figs 16.3A and B) are almost same as that of duodenum except in few places where jejunum shows:

- Mucosal villi are rich in mucus secreting goblet cells and along with submucosa they form prominent circular folds called **plicae circularis** or **valves of kerkring**.
- Small region of submucosa containing loose areolar connective tissue and absence of Brunner's glands.

Discussions

- Name the four layers of jejunum.
- What is plicae circularis?
- Where do you see intestinal glands in jejunum?
- List the histological differences between duodenum and jejunum.

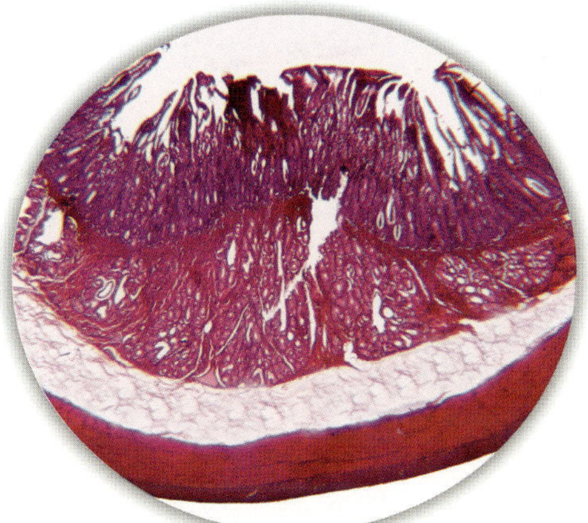

A

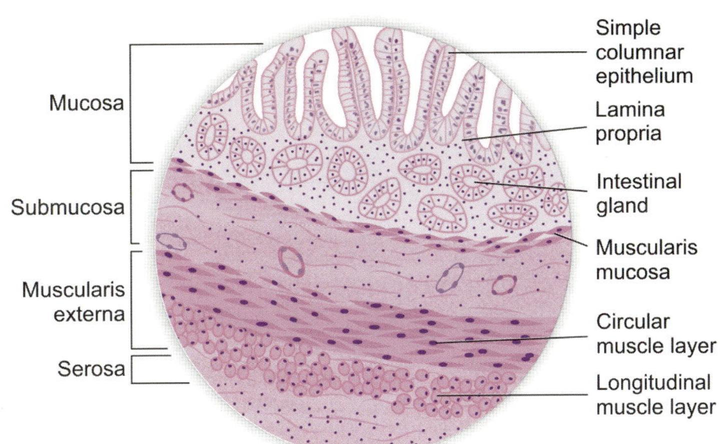

B

Figures 16.3A and B: Jejunum [transverse section (TS)]. **A.** Photograph; **B.** Diagrammatic representation.

ILEUM (TS)

Slide No. 38

Identification Points

- Small villi rich in goblet cells
- Crypts of Lieberkühn present
- Mucosa containing Peyer's patches.

Structure

Histological features of ileum (Figs 16.4A and B) can be explained as follows:

Mucosa: It is lined by simple columnar epithelium. Here villi are very small and lamina propria contains few intestinal glands and numerous aggregations of lymphatic nodules called **Peyer's patches**. Muscularis mucosa is disrupted here.

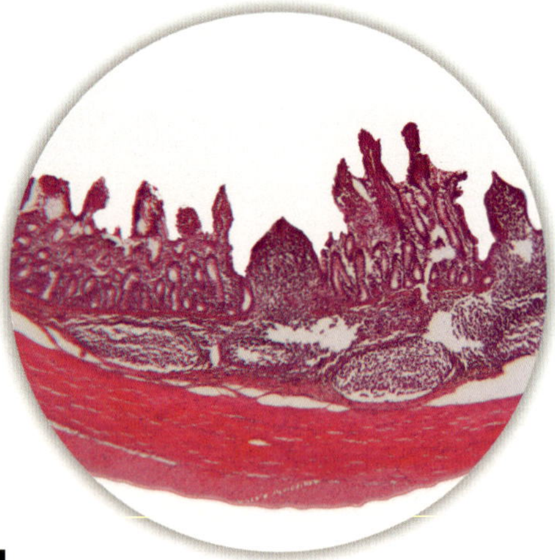

A

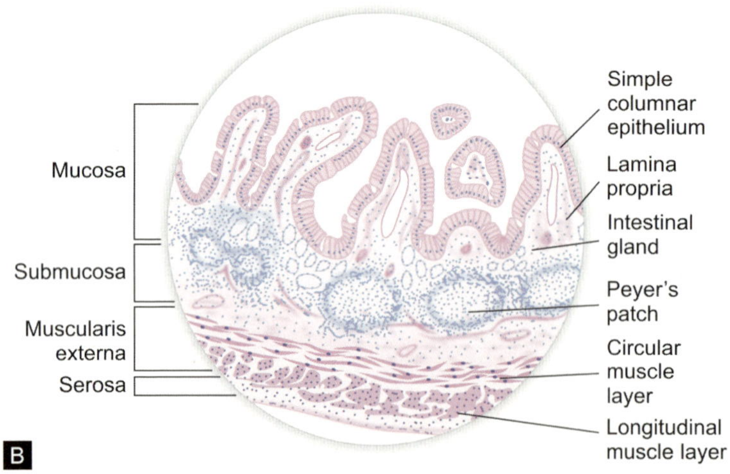

B

Figures 16.4A and B: Ileum [transverse section (TS)]. **A.** Photograph; **B.** Diagrammatic representation.

Submucosa: It is very thin and small, made up of loose areolar connective tissue. It also contains some lymphoid tissue, which is migrated from lamina propria.

Muscularis externa: It is made up of thin layer of inner circular and outer longitudinal muscle fibers.

Serosa: Contains connective tissue cells with a layer of visceral peritoneum.

Discussions

- Name the different layers of ileum.
- What are Peyer's patches?
- List the differences between jejunum and ileum.

VERMIFORM APPENDIX (TS)

Slide No. 39

Identification Points

- Villi are absent
- Lamina propria containing lymphoid aggregations
- Thick muscular layer.

Introduction

Vermiform appendix (Figs 16.5A and B) is a worm like diverticulum arising from posteromedial wall of cecum.

Structure

Histological features of vermiform appendix are as follows.

Mucosa: It is the innermost layer lined by simple columnar epithelium with many goblet cells in it:

- Villi are almost absent in mucosa and few intestinal glands are seen in lamina propria of appendix.
- In between the glands their exists many lymphoid aggregations, which extend into submucosa.
- Here the muscularis mucosa is disrupted.

Submucosa: It is made up of loose areolar connective tissue with many blood vessels in it. It also contains the lymphoid tissue migrated from lamina propria.

Muscularis externa: It is made up of inner circular and outer longitudinal muscle fibers with myenteric nerve plexus in between.

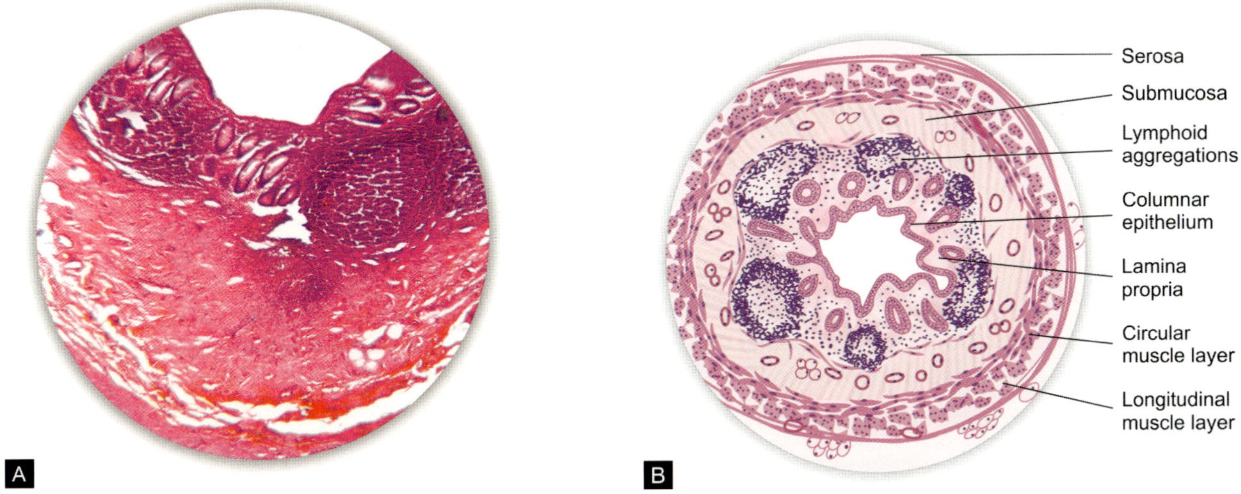

Figures 16.5A and B: Vermiform appendix [transverse section (TS)]. **A.** Photograph; **B.** Diagrammatic representation.

Serosa: It is the outermost layer of appendix associated with few adipocytes.

- Vermiform appendix is said to be rudimentary in nature hence it does not perform any function in the human body.

Clinical Histology

Inflammation of the vermiform appendix is called **appendicitis**. It is caused either by obstruction (impact of hard stool in the lumen) or by infections.

Surgical removal of vermiform appendix is termed as **appendicectomy.**

Discussions

- Where is vermiform appendix located?
- Name the layers of vermiform appendix and which layer is more prominent?
- Are villi seen in vermiform appendix?
- Explain the muscularis externa of vermiform appendix.
- What is appendicitis?
- What is appendicectomy?

LARGE INTESTINE (COLON TS)

Slide No. 40

Identification Points

- Mucosa with folds, but no villi
- Numerous goblets cells
- Prominent tenia coli.

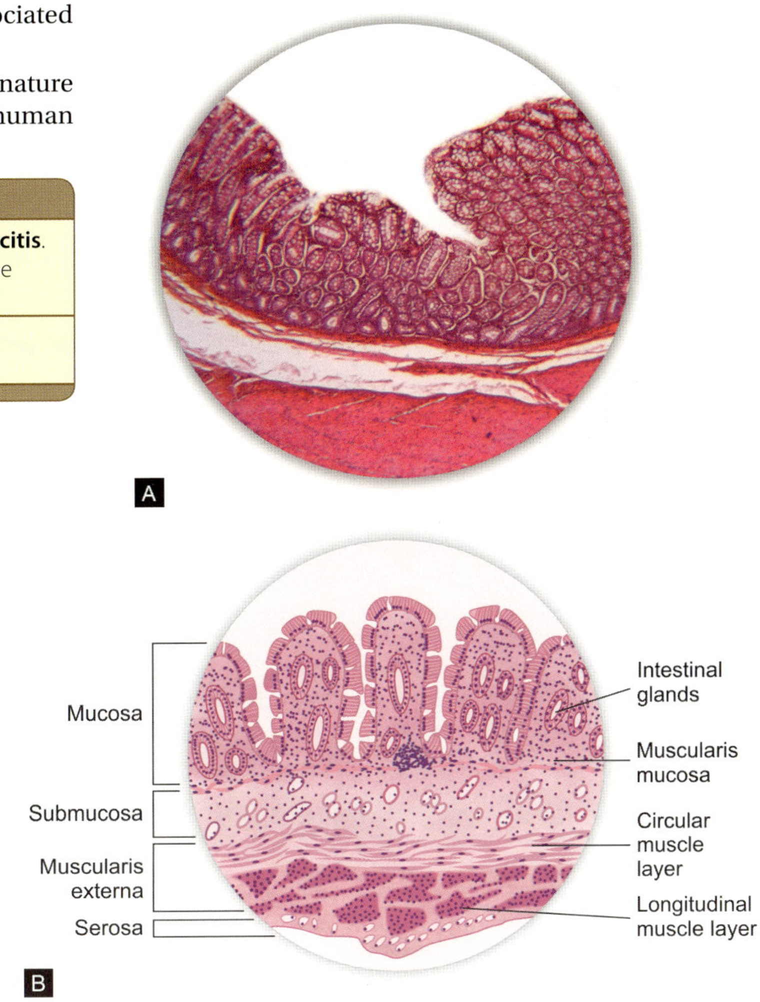

Figures 16.6A and B: Large intestine [transverse section (TS)]. **A.** Photograph; **B.** Diagrammatic representation.

Structure

A transverse section of large intestine (Figs 16.6A and B) shows following features.

Mucosa: It is lined by simple columnar epithelium rich in mucus secreting goblet cells. Here mucosa does not contain villi.

Just below the mucosa there are numerous intestinal glands (crypts of Lieberkühn) distributed within the lamina propria, however, it does not contain Paneth cells.

Submucosa: It is made up of loose areolar connective tissue cells and fibers with numerous adipocytes in it.

Muscularis externa: It consists of inner circular and outer longitudinal muscle layer.

- In certain regions of colon longitudinal muscle layers becomes very thick resulting in formation of three band like structures called **Tenia coli**.

Serosa: It is said to be incomplete in posterior aspect of ascending and descending colon. Here it shows many peritoneal pockets filled with adipose tissue and is termed as **appendices epiploicae**.

Discussions

- Name the different layers of colon.
- Name the surface epithelium lining the mucosa of colon?
- Where do you see crypts of Lieberkühn?
- What are tenia coli?
- What is appendices epiploicae?

PANCREAS (Figs 16.7A and B)

Slide No. 41

Identification Points

- Numerous serous acini
- Islets of Langerhans are present
- Interlobular ducts are seen.

Introduction

- Pancreas is a J-shaped organ situated in posterior abdominal wall.
- It is divided into head, neck, body and tail, where head is fitted in the curve of duodenum and tail is pointed towards the hilum of spleen.

Structure

Histology of spleen shows following different features.

Capsule: The pancreas is thin, made up of dense irregular connective tissue.

- Connective tissue septae of the capsule enters the parenchyma of the gland and divides the whole parenchyma into numerous lobules.

Parenchyma: Here parenchyma of the gland is said to be distinct from other glands as it contains both exocrine and endocrine glandular cells in it. Therefore, pancreas is said to be a **heterocrine gland.**

Exocrine part: This comprises about 70%–80% of the total parenchyma of the gland.

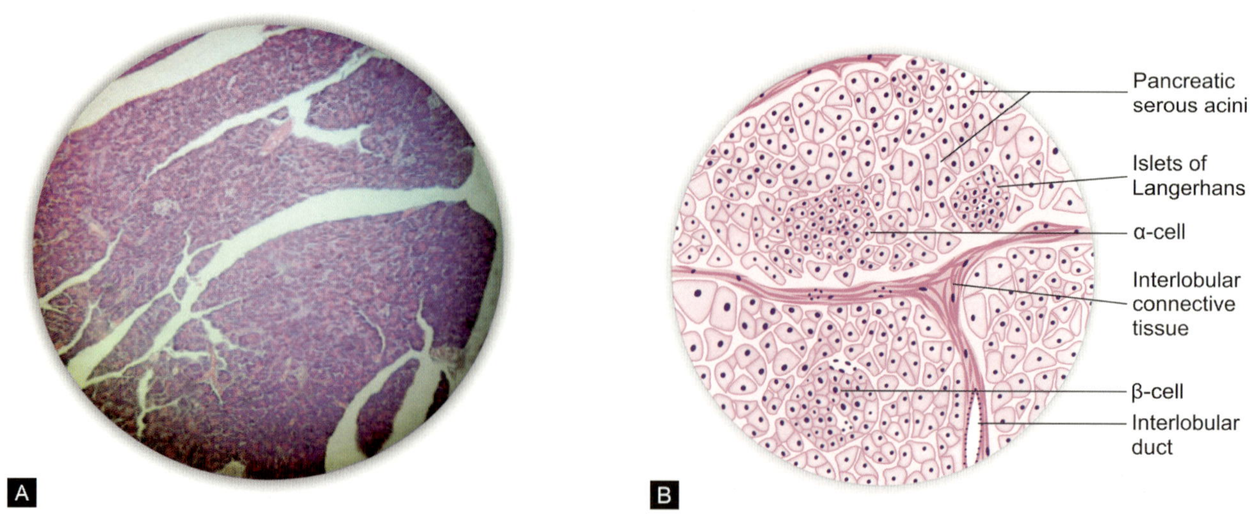

Figures 16.7A and B: Pancreas. **A.** Photograph; **B.** Diagrammatic representation.

- It is made up of numerous serous acini with a smaller lumen (for more details refer the histology of parotid gland).

Functions

Serous acini of exocrine pancreas secrete pancreatic juice and many digestive enzymes.

- Pancreatic juice is an alkaline fluid, which plays an important role in neutralization of acid chyme thus aiding the process of digestion whereas pancreatic enzymes act on protein, fat and carbohydrate food substances and convert them into simpler molecules for their easy absorption from the gut.

Endocrine part: This comprises about 20%–30% of the total parenchyma of the gland.

- Endocrine part of the gland is predominately well-developed in the tail region and it consists of aggregations of numerous cells forming many clusters, which are referred to as **Islets of Langerhans.**

The different types of cells present in Islets of Langerhans are:

- α-cells (A-cells)
- β-cells (B-cells)
- δ-cells (D-cells).

α-cells: They constitute about 25% of the endocrine pancreas.

- They are peripherally situated in the Islets of Langerhans and can be identified by their small size and pink cytoplasm.

β-cells: They constitute about 70% of the total cell population in endocrine pancreas.

- They are the large cells with blue cytoplasm and are situated more at the center of the islets.

δ-cells: These cells constitute hardly about 5% of the endocrine pancreas.

- They are highly variable in their size and can occur anywhere in the Islets of Langerhans.
- Though they are present in the Islet of Langerhans, they are not usually demonstrated because of its less population and variable size.

Functions

- α-cells secrete a hormone called **glucagon,** which converts the excess glycogen into glucose thus increasing the blood glucose level.
- β-cells secrete a hormone called **insulin** which converts the excess glucose into glycogen thus decreasing the blood glucose level to normal.
- δ-cell probably produces few local hormones like **gastrin, somatostatin and vasoactive intestinal polypeptide (VIP),** which produce local effect on gastrointestinal tract.

Clinical Histology

Inflammation of the exocrine pancreas is termed as **pancreatitis.**

Diabetes mellitus is an endocrine disorder characterized by increased blood glucose level in the blood due to pathology in endocrine pancreas.

It is either due to hyposecretion of insulin by B-cells or due to destruction of receptors for insulin hormone.

Discussions

- Why is pancreas a heterocrine gland?
- Describe the exocrine part of pancreas.
- Which type of cells form the exocrine pancreas?
- What are Islets of Langerhans?
- List the different cells of Islets of Langerhans with one function each.
- List the functions of exocrine and endocrine pancreas.
- What is pancreatitis?
- What is diabetes mellitus? Why is it due to?

CHAPTER

17 Hepatobiliary System

INTRODUCTION

- Hepatobiliary system is an important system of the body, which is responsible for the synthesis, transportation, storage and concentration of the bile and its constituents. The organs involved are liver and gallbladder.
- Even though it is a part of digestive system, recent advances and researches have recognized the importance of liver and gallbladder, which made pathologists and histologists to consider it as **hepatobiliary system**.

LIVER

Slide No. 42

Identification Points

- Hepatic lobules with central vein
- Radiating hepatic cord cells
- Portal triad.

Introduction

- Liver is the largest exocrine gland situated mainly in the right hypochondrium and a part of left hypochondrium in abdomen (Figs 17.1A and B).
- It has two lobes, the bigger right lobe and a smaller left lobe. Both the lobes are separated by **falciform ligament**.
- Development of liver starts in **4th** week of intrauterine life; it arises from the caudal end of foregut as a hepatic bud, which later grows as **pars hepatica** to form liver.

Structure

Structure can be explained under following headings.

Capsule: Apart from peritoneum, liver is also covered by a thin layer of connective tissue called **Glisson's capsule**. This capsule surrounds the liver and hepatic blood vessels thus enter the liver through porta hepatis, which in turn divides the whole liver into numerous lobules.

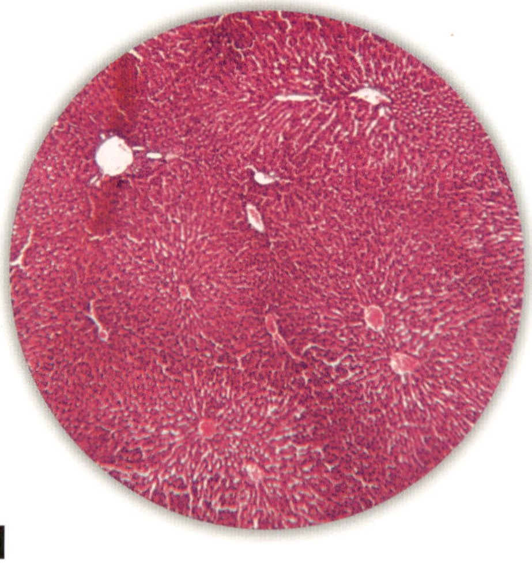

A

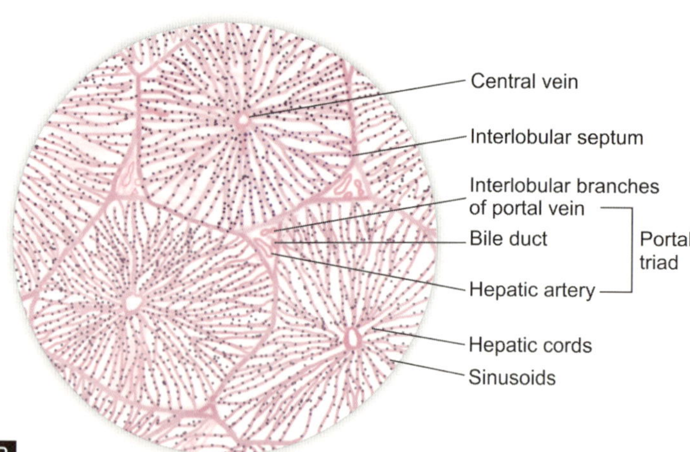

B

Figures 17.1A and B: Liver. **A.** Photograph; **B.** Diagrammatic representation.

Stroma: It consists of thin layer of **reticular fibers** surrounding the hepatic cord cells and sinusoids. It acts like framework of the liver by supporting the liver cells and sinusoids.

Parenchyma: A repeated units of hepatic lobules form the whole of the liver parenchyma, which is explained as follows.

Hepatic lobule: It is a microscopic area of the liver, which is hexagonal/polygonal in shape and is covered by a thin connective tissue septum called **interlobular septum.**

- There is a **central vein** at the center of the hepatic lobule and hepatic cord cells are radiating from the central vein.
- The hepatic cord cells are hexagonal-shaped cells with central prominent nucleus and well-developed cell organelles in it. These cells are also known as **hepatocytes**. They are arranged in the form of plates that branch and anastomose with one another to form a network-like structure.
- On an average 85%–90% of the liver parenchyma is made up of hepatocytes and 10%–15% of it is formed by sinusoidal epithelium.
- In between the two layers of hepatic cord cells there are sinusoids made up of **fenestrated endothelium and von Kupffer cells**.
- von Kupffer cells act as macrophages and destruct the old red blood cells (RBCs), thus form a part of reticuloendothelial system.

Bile canaliculi: In the microscopic view of liver, each hepatocyte is connected to another hepatocyte by the extension of cytoplasmic threads, which pass through the minute canals of the matrix and are called **Bile canaliculi**.

Perisinusoidal space of dissae: It is a minute potential space found in between the endothelium of sinusoids and hepatic cord cells. It contains:

- **Reticular fibers**.
- **Microvilli** of hepatic cord cells.
- **Perisinusoidal lipocytes/ITO cells/Stellate cells.**
  - ITO cells are rich in fat with vitamin A and secrete intralobular matrix including reticular fibers.

Space of mall: The blood vessels and hepatic ducts present in portal canals are surrounded by a narrow interval space called **Space of mall**.

Portal canal: It is an interval space found in between the hepatic lobules and is filled by connective tissue. It contains portal triad in it.

Portal triad: It contains an interlobular branch of hepatic artery, an interlobular branch of portal vein and an interlobular bile duct (Figs 17.2A and B).

Portal lobule: It is the **true functional unit of the liver**, where a single branch of portal vein supplies the three adjoining hepatic lobules (Fig. 17.3).

Portal acinus: It is a diamond-shaped area found in between two central veins of the hepatic lobule, where the corners of the diamond are formed by the hepatic triad. Based on the blood supply to this area it is divided in to three zones.

Zone 1: It is that part of the liver, which is close to the arterial and portal blood vessels and it has got good blood supply.

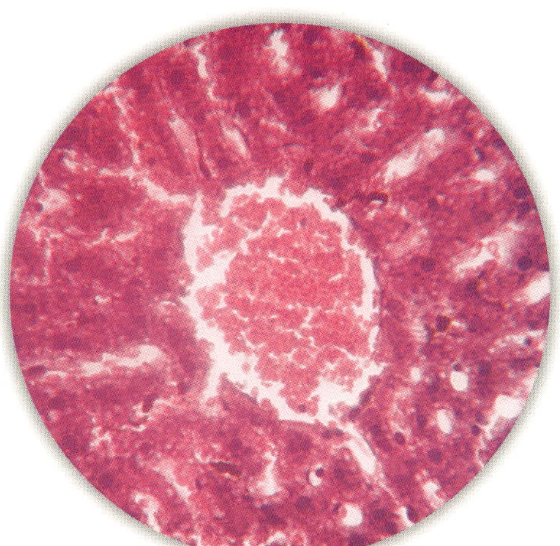

A

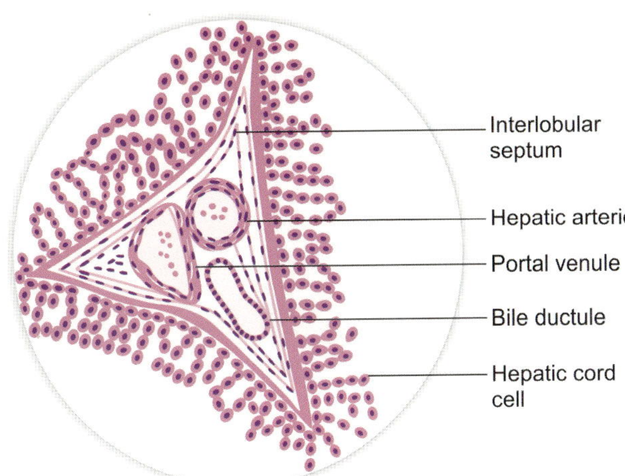

B

Figures 17.2A and B: A. Central vein with radiating hepatic cord cells; **B.** Diagrammatic view of portal triad.

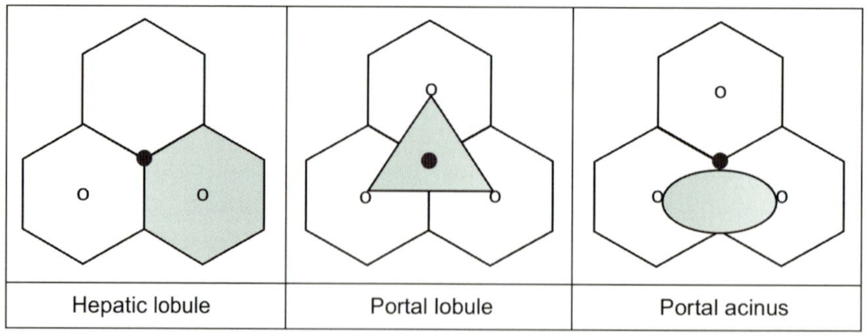

Figure 17.3: Different important areas of liver

Zone 2: It is an intermediate area found in between zone 1 and zone 3 and it has got moderate blood supply.

Zone 3: The area of hepatic cord cells surrounding the central vein forms zone 3 and it has got poor blood supply.

Functions

- Active site of metabolism of carbohydrate, proteins, lipids, vitamins, drugs and many hormones.
- **Glycogenesis:** Conversion of glucose to glycogen.
- **Glycogenolysis:** Conversion of glycogen to glucose.
- **Gluconeogenesis:** Conversion of amino acids into glucose.
- Secretes bile juice.
- Excretes bile pigments, heavy metals, cholesterol, toxins, etc.

Clinical Histology
Hepatomegaly is a condition where there is increase in the size of liver and is seen in fatty liver
Jaundice is the common disease of liver, characterized by altered liver functions and increased bilirubin level in blood
Viral infection of the liver is called **hepatitis** and the viruses affecting are Hepatitis—A, B, C, D and E
Intracellular accumulation of neutral fat in hepatocytes leads to **fatty liver**
Cirrhosis of liver is a condition where the normal lobular structure of hepatic parenchyma is affected with necrosis and fibrosis
Amebic liver abscess is a liver disorder caused by a protozoan parasite *Entamoeba histolytica,* which is characterized by the abscess formation in liver cells
In **chronic venous congestion** of liver zone 3 cells are severally affected

- Chief organ of heat production.
- Site of hemopoiesis in fetal life.
- Forms a part of **reticuloendothelial system**.
- Acts as detoxification center.
- Produces plasma proteins and blood clotting factors.
- Stores fat-soluble vitamins such as A, D, E, K, iron, folic acid, etc.

Discussions

- What is Glisson's capsule?
- What are bile canaliculi?
- What is portal triad?
- What is the function of von Kupffer cell?
- What is space of disease and what does it contain?
- What is LTO cell and what is its function?
- List the functions of liver.
- What is space of mall?
- What is fatty liver?
- What is jaundice?
- What is cirrhosis of liver?
- What is hepatitis?

GALLBLADDER

Slide No. 43

Identification Points

- Honeycomb appearance of mucosa
- Absence of submucosa and muscularis mucosa
- Presence of fibromuscular coat.

Introduction

- Gallbladder is a muscular sac-like structure situated in fossa of gallbladder (visceral surface of liver) (Figs 17.4A and B).

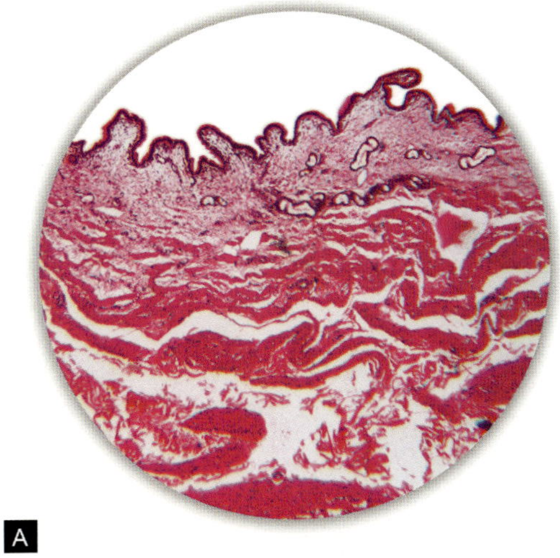

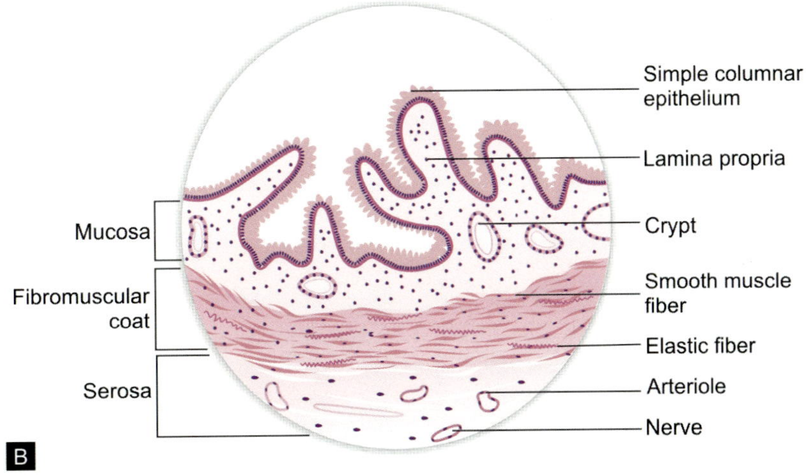

Figures 17.4A and B: Gallbladder. **A.** Photograph; **B.** Diagrammatic representation.

- Different parts of the gallbladder are fundus, body and neck.
- In **4th** week of intrauterine life gallbladder develops from **pars cystica,** which is a part of hepatic bud.

Structure

A histological feature of the gallbladder shows following layers.

Mucosa: It is the inner-most layer of the gallbladder lined by simple columnar epithelial cells and a thin layer of lamina propria underneath it:

- These cells bear numerous **microvilli** at its tip and goblet cells are absent.
- Mucosa of gallbladder is highly folded forming many rugae giving rise to **honeycomb appearance**.
- Here submucosa and muscularis mucosal layers are absent.

Fibromuscular layers: It is seen just beneath the lamina propria, which consists of circularly arranged smooth muscle cells with few elastic fibers in it.

Serosa: It is the outermost layer of gallbladder made up of dense irregular connective tissue with few blood vessels in it.

Functions

- Stores bile.
- Concentrates the bile.
- Decreases the pH of bile.
- Concentration capacity of gallbladder maintains the pressure in the biliary system, which is essential for the release of bile into small intestine.

Clinical Histology
Inflammation of the gallbladder is called **cholecystitis**
Surgical removal of the gallbladder is called **cholecystectomy**
Formation of gallstones in gallbladder results in **cholelithiasis**

Discussions

- What is the location of gallbladder?
- What is the normal color of gallbladder?
- What do you mean by honeycomb appearance of gallbladder?
- Name the layers of gallbladder.
- Which two layers are absent in gallbladder?
- List the functions of gallbladder.
- What is the function of cholecystokinin?
- What is cholecystitis?
- What is cholelithiasis?
- What is cholecystectomy?

CHAPTER 18

Renal System

INTRODUCTION

- Urinary system is one of the important systems, which clean the body by removing unwanted and toxic substances from blood.
- Even though skin and lungs are also said to perform the same function, but the major role is played by the renal system, which includes kidney, ureter, urinary bladder and urethra.
- Let us know the basic structural and functional unit of kidney to know more about its histology.

NEPHRON

- Nephron is the structural and functional unit of kidney (Fig. 18.1)
- On an average each kidney consists of about 1 million of nephrons.

Structure

Nephron is divided into two main parts:
- Renal corpuscles.
- Renal tubules.

Renal corpuscle is made up of glomerulus and Bowman's capsule; whereas renal tubule includes different tubules like proximal convoluted tubule, loop of Henle and distal convoluted tubule.

Renal Corpuscle

Glomerulus: It is a tuft of capillaries placed in the cavity of Bowman's capsule:

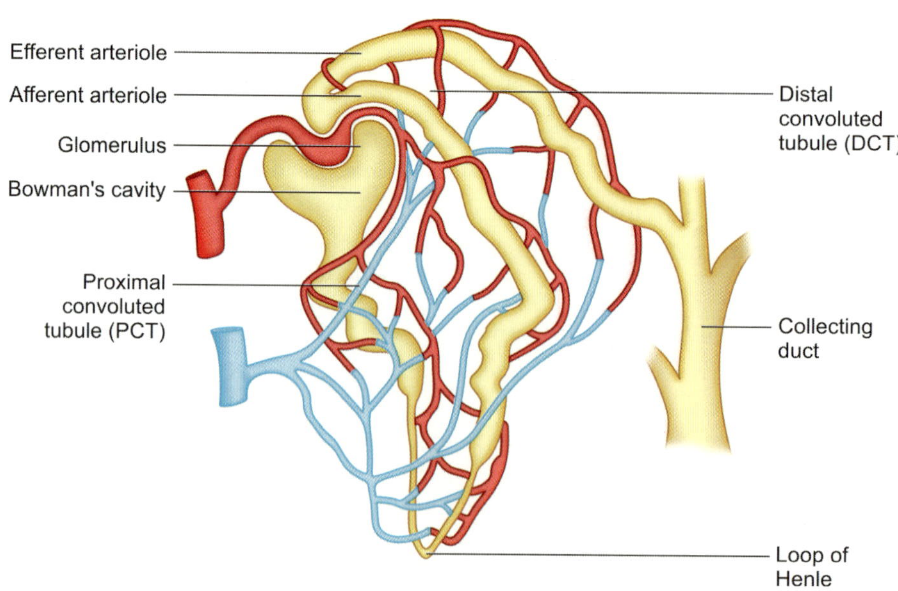

Figure 18.1: Nephron

- It consists of an afferent arteriole, which enters the Bowman's cavity, divides rapidly forming a tuft of capillary and emerges out as an efferent arteriole
- Always the diameter of afferent arteriole is greater than that of diameter of efferent arteriole, which is very essential for the production of glomerular filtration rate (GFR).

Function

Glomerulus is responsible for the generation of **GFR,** i.e. filtration of the substances from the blood of glomerulus into the capsular spaces of Bowman's capsule through endothelial capsular membranes under high ultrafiltration pressure.

Bowman's capsule: It is a cup-shaped structure, which encloses a tuft of capillaries in it and the space present in it is called **Bowman's space.**

- Bowman's capsule is made up of two layers—an outer parietal layer and an inner visceral layer
- Both the layers are lined by modified simple squamous epithelium, which is resting on basement membrane; but the visceral layer epithelium bears numerous feet, like processes called **pedicles** through which it is attached to the basement membrane and such cells are called **podocytes.**

Function

Collection and storage of ultrafiltrate takes place in Bowman's capsule and the filtrate is called **primary urine.**

Renal Tubule

Proximal convoluted tubule: It is a thick tubule arising as the continuation of Bowman's capsule and is located in cortex of kidney.

- Since it is highly convoluted and is proximal to the renal corpuscles, hence it is called **proximal convoluted tubule (PCT)**
- The internal surface of PCT is lined by brush-bordered cuboidal epithelium, which increases the area of absorption.

Function

Proximal convoluted tubule is absorptive in function. It selectively absorbs monosaccharides, amino acids, fatty acids and glycerol molecules present in the primary urine.

Loop of Henle: It is the continuation of PCT, which lies in the medulla of kidney. It consists of a long thick descending limb lined by brush-bordered cuboidal epithelium and a short thin ascending limb lined by simple squamous epithelium.

Function

Loop of Henle generates a gradual increase in the osmotic gradient in the interstitium of medulla by **counter current mechanism.** This helps in absorption of sodium and water.

Distal convoluted tubule: It is a thick segment or tubule arising as the continuation of the ascending loop of Henle.

- It has a small straight part with large distal convoluted part hence the name **distal convoluted tubule (DCT)**
- A small part of DCT lies in medulla and rest of the major portion of DCT is located in cortex of kidney
- Histologically, distal convoluted tubule is lined by simple cuboidal epithelium with no brush borders.

Functions

- The process of reabsorption takes place within DCT with a small amount of water absorption.
- It is also secretary in function and secretes potassium ions and other waste (toxic) substances into the tubular lumen.

Collecting Duct

- Collecting duct is a large duct, which is formed by the union of many DCTs
- It is lined by simple columnar epithelium and is located in both cortex and medulla.

Juxtaglomerular Apparatus

Juxtaglomerular apparatus is a specialized tissue situated near the glomerulus of each nephron.

It is made up of:

- Juxtaglomerular (JG) cells
- Macula densa of DCT
- Extraglomerular mesangial cells or lacis cells.

The cells of juxtaglomerular apparatus belong to APUD cell system (APUD stands for 'amine precursor uptake decarboxylase').

Functions

- Juxtaglomerular apparatus secretes renin, which undergoes a complex series of reactions finally causing:
  - Maintenance of GFR.
  - Stimulation of adrenal cortex to secrete aldosterone.
  - Regulation of renal blood pressure.

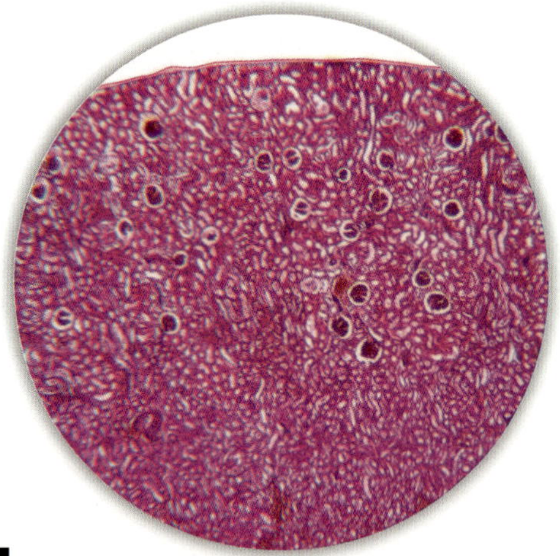

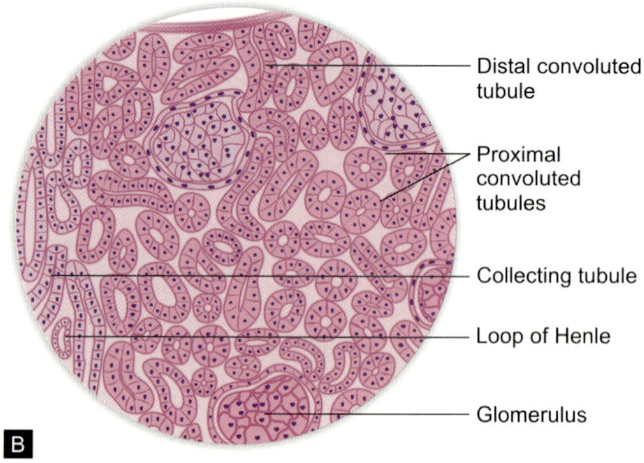

Figures 18.2A and B: Section of kidney. **A.** Photograph; **B.** Diagrammatic representation.

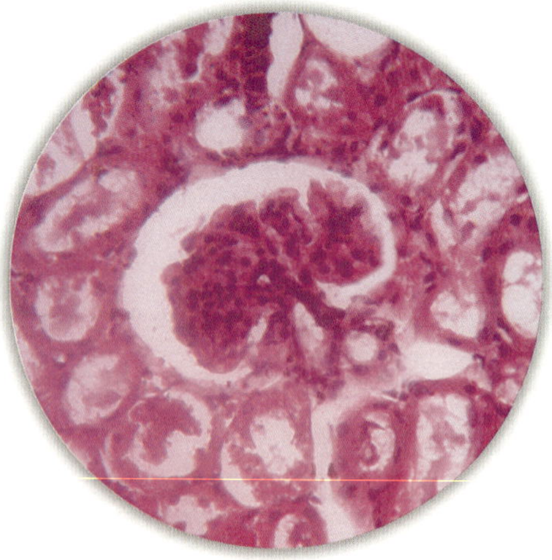

Figure 18.3: Glomerulus

KIDNEY (Figs 18.2A and B, 18.3)

Slide No. 44

Identification Points

- Outer cortex and inner medulla
- Cortex containing renal corpuscles, proximal and distal convoluted tubules
- Medulla containing Henle's loop and collecting ducts.

Introduction

Kidney is a pair of excretory organ located in the posterior abdominal wall behind the peritoneum.

Structure

Capsule: It is the outermost protective covering made up of dense irregular connective tissue. External to it there is condensation of peripheral fat as perinephric pad of fat which, in turn, is surrounded by a sheath called renal fascia.

Cortex: It is the outer part of kidney found just below the capsule. It mainly contains glomerulus, Bowman's capsule, DCTs near by it and few PCTs also. The features of these structures are same as explained in previous discussions.

Medulla: It is the inner part of kidney found below the cortex. Medulla is rich in loop of Henle, collecting tubules and **papillary ducts (ducts of Bellini).**

Clinical Histology
Nephrotic syndrome is a disease of kidney characterized by the massive proteinuria, hypoalbuminemia and edema
Inflammation of the glomerulus leads degenerative changes in glomerulus called **glomerulonephritis**
Failure of kidney to perform its function or inability of the kidney to maintain the homeostasis of blood and body fluids is known as **renal failure**

Discussions

- Name the different parts of kidney.
- What is nephron?
- What are the different parts of nephron?
- Name the epithelium lining seen in:
  - PCT.
  - Loop of Henle.

  - DCT.
  - Collecting duct.
- What is the function of following?
  - PCT.
  - Loop of Henle.
  - DCT.
- What is diabetes insipidus?
- What is renal failure?

URETER (TS) (Figs 18.4A to C)

Slide No. 45

Identification Points

- Star-shaped lumen
- Mucosa lined by transitional epithelium
- Inner longitudinal and outer circular muscle coat present.

Introduction

Ureter is a muscular tube-like structure, which connects the kidney to urinary bladder.

Structure

A transverse section of ureter can be explained by the following.

Mucosa: It is the innermost layer of ureter lined by transitional epithelium with lamina propria underneath it. Mucosa of ureter is thrown into many folds, which give a star-shaped appearance to the lumen and it is one of the important identification points in TS of ureter.

Muscular layer: It is found just below the lamina propria.

- It consists of an inner longitudinal muscle layer and outer circular muscle layer

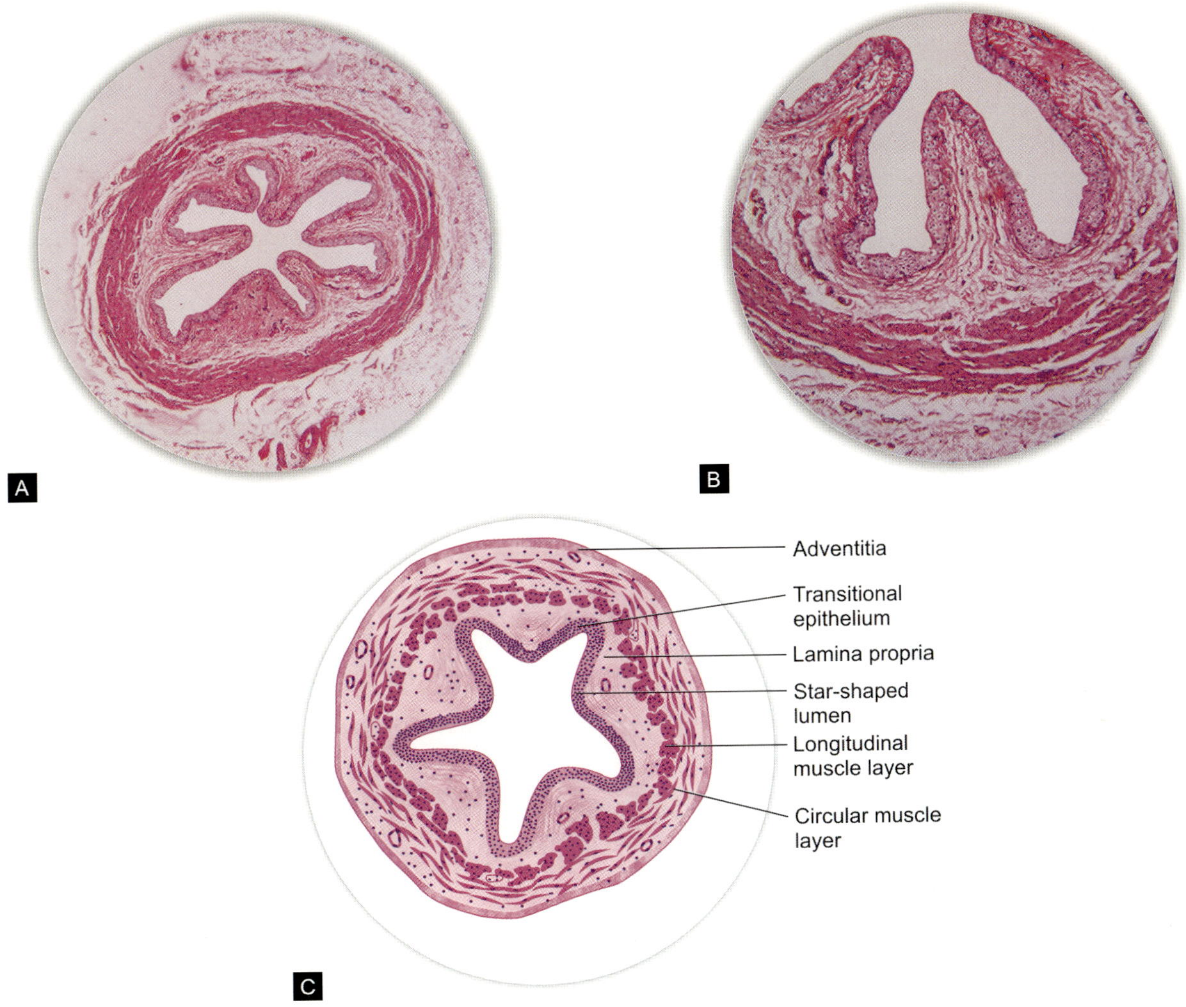

Figures 18.4A to C: Ureter [transverse section (TS)]. **A and B.** Photographs; **C.** Diagrammatic representation.

- Apart from this the lower one third of ureter contains an additional layer of longitudinal muscles.

Adventitia: It is the outermost protective covering layer made up of dense irregular connective tissue.

Functions

- Transitional epithelium lining of the ureter prevents the entry of urine and its toxic substances into the blood vessels of ureter by diffusion.
- Muscular layer is responsible for the peristalsis in ureter, which pushes the urine from kidney to urinary bladder.
- Adventitia is protective and supportive in function.

Clinical Histology

Formation of stones in kidney and its other parts is known as renal calculi and is more common in ureter. It is characterized by an intense colic pain in the loin.

Discussions

- Name the epithelium lining the ureter.
- What is the importance of lumen in identifying the ureter?
- Name the different layers of ureter.
- Enumerate the functions of different layers of ureter.
- What is kinking of ureter?
- What are renal calculi?

URINARY BLADDER (Figs 18.5A and B)

Slide No. 46

Identification Points

- Mucosa lined by transitional epithelium
- Submucosa is absent
- Muscular layer containing detrusor muscles.

Introduction

- Urinary bladder is a muscular bag-like structure, which temporarily stores urine for voiding
- Its normal storing capacity is about 200–300 mL.

Structure

Structure of urinary bladder can be explained as follows.

Mucosa: It is the innermost layer of urinary bladder lined by transitional epithelium with a lamina propria rich in blood vessels underneath it.

- The mucosa is thrown into many folds, which expand to collect more quantity of urine with- in the bladder.

Muscular layer: This layer of urinary bladder is not well-defined and it is said to be almost irregular, consisting of inner longitudinal, middle circular and outer longitudinal muscle layer.

- Few muscles fibers around the internal ureteric orifices form an internal urethral sphincter, which control the outflow of urine from the bladder.

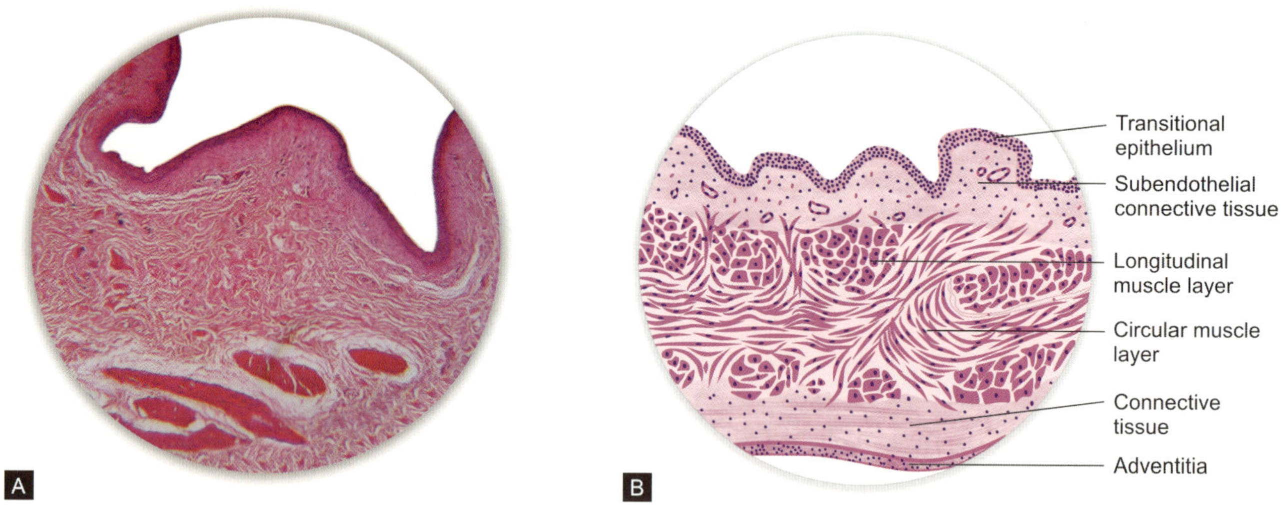

Figures 18.5A and B: Urinary bladder [transverse section (TS)]. **A.** Photograph; **B.** Diagrammatic representation.

Adventitia: This is an outermost layer of urinary bladder made up of dense irregular connective tissue and partly by serosa.

Functions

- Transitional epithelium lining of the mucosa prevents the entry of urine and its toxic substances into the urinary bladder tissue. Here the cells also decrease in size and layers to accommodate large quantity of urine.
- The prominent muscular coat is responsible for the micturition process by producing the powerful contractions.
- Adventitia is protective and supportive in nature.

Clinical Histology

Usually the transitional epithelium lining the urinary bladder is 4–6 cell layers thick. If it increases more than 6 cell layers thickness, then it is suggestive of carcinoma of urinary bladder.

Discussions

- List the different layers in urinary bladder.
- Name the epithelium lining the mucosa of urinary bladder. What is its significance?
- Enumerate the functions of different layers of urinary bladder.
- Name a histological indication of carcinoma urinary bladder.

Chapter

19 Respiratory System

INTRODUCTION

- Respiratory system is one of the important systems in body, which is necessary for oxygenation of the body cells.
- Respiratory system is divided into two parts—upper and lower respiratory tract.
- Anything above the vocal cords belongs to upper respiratory tract and below it belongs to lower respiratory tract.

CLASSIFICATION (Fig. 19.1)

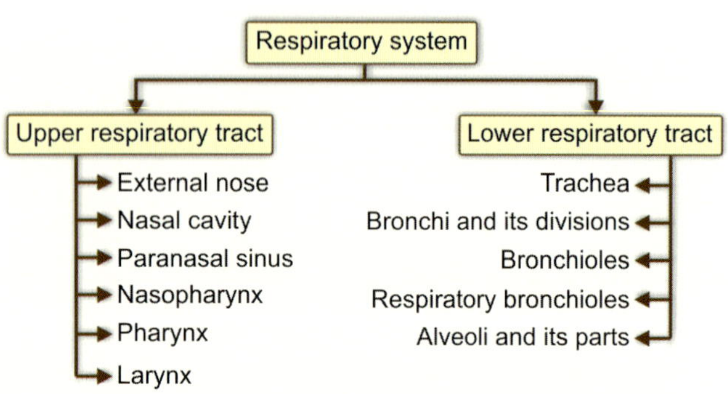

Figure 19.1: Classification of respiratory system

FUNCTIONS

Respiratory Functions

- Respiration helps in providing oxygen from lungs to different parts of the body.
- It also removes unwanted gases (CO_2, CO, NO) from different parts of the body back to environment through lungs.

Non-respiratory Functions

- Olfactory receptors present in the nasal mucosa are responsible for olfaction.
- Pseudostratified ciliated columnar epithelium lining the upper respiratory tract prevents the entry of foreign dust particles and other microorganisms into the system.
- Vocal cords of larynx are responsible for the productions of voice.
- Different types of phagocytic cells present in lung tissue provide defense to the body.
- Regulation of body water, body temperature and acid-base balance is also an important function of respiratory system.

TRACHEA (TS)

Slide No. 47

Identification Points

- Mucosa lined by pseudostratified ciliated columnar epithelium with goblet cells
- Submucosa containing serous and mucous glands
- Hyaline cartilaginous ring.

Introduction

- Trachea (Figs 19.2A and B) is a part of lower respiratory tract, which extends from lower border of cricoid cartilage up to the level of sternal angle.
- Since it is a hollow tubular structure through which air passes in hence, it is also called **windpipe.**
- Trachea is supported by 15–20 C-shaped cartilaginous rings throughout its course for maintaining its lumen patency.

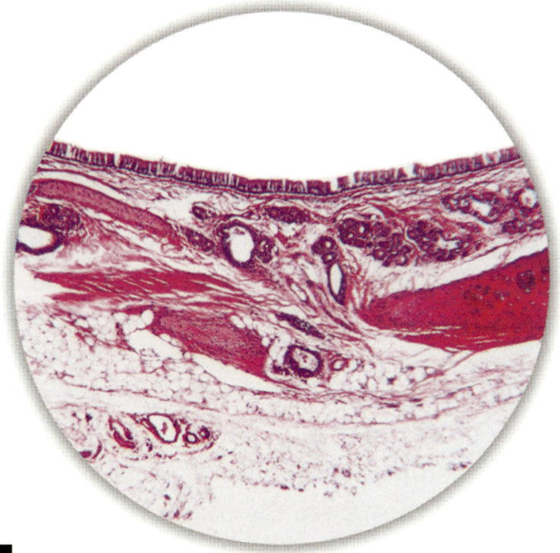

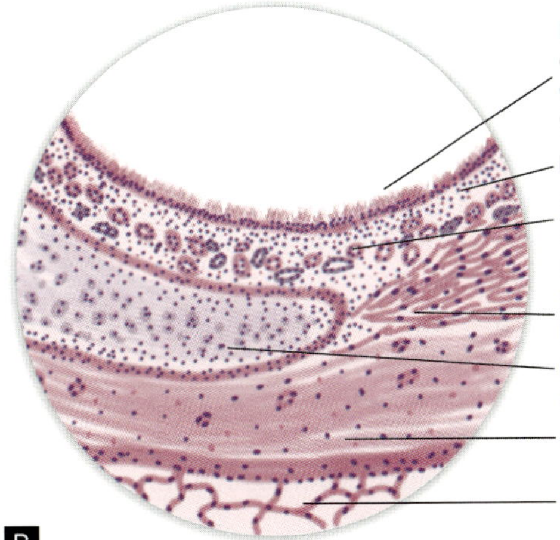

Figures 19.2A and B: Trachea [transverse section (TS)]. **A.** Photograph; **B.** Diagrammatic representation.

Structure

Structure can be explained under following headings.

Mucosa: It is lined by a layer of pseudostratified ciliated columnar epithelium with lots of goblet cells in between. Just below the epithelium there is lamina propria rich in elastic fibers and lymphocytes with few mast cells in it.

Submucosa: It is made up of loose areolar connective tissue with blood capillaries in it. Along with few lymphoid tissues, mass of serous and mucous glands are also seen in submucosa.

Cartilaginous layer: It is made up of C-shaped hyaline cartilage with few smooth muscles and fibroelastic tissue, which connects free ends of the cartilage.

Adventitia: It is rich in fibroelastic tissue with few blood vessels in it.

Functions

- Pseudostratified ciliated columnar epithelium lining the mucosa performs ciliary action thus prevents the entry of dust particles into respiratory system.
- Serous glands present in submucosa keep the epithelium moist and prevent the infection whereas mucous glands secrete thick mucus, which covers the epithelial lining and helps in trapping dust.
- Cartilaginous ring is responsible for the maintenance of normal patency of the tracheal lumen.
- Adventitia layer is protective and supportive in function.

Clinical Histology
Immotile cilia syndrome is a syndrome characterized by the immotility of cilia of the respiratory tract epithelial lining leading to bronchiectasis
Improper secretion of serous glands may lead to dryness of epithelial surfaces finally causing acute infections like acute bronchitis
Bronchial asthma is a respiratory disorder characterized by spasmodic contraction of tracheal smooth muscles with increased mucus secretion ultimately blocking the air passage

Discussions

- What is the another name for trachea? Why is it called so?
- How many cartilaginous rings support the tracheal framework?
- Name the muscle and ligament, which connects the two free ends of the cartilaginous ring.
- Name the layers of trachea with one function each.
- List the functions of trachea.
- What is bronchial asthma?

LUNG

Slide No. 48

Identification Points

- Honey comb appearance of alveoli
- Simple squamous epithelium lining the pulmonary alveoli

- Intrapulmonary bronchi, bronchioles and respiratory bronchioles are seen.

Introduction

- Lungs (Figs 19.3A and B) are the pair of respiratory organs placed in a protective thoracic cage. Here right lung has three lobes whereas left lung has got two lobes and right lung is slightly bigger than the left.
- Development of lung starts in the **4th week** of intrauterine life as a tracheal bud (tracheobronchial primordium). This **tracheal bud** grows in size against the pleura thus finally differentiating into different components of lung tissue with a protective covering of double-layered pleura.

Structure

A detailed structure of lung tissue can be explained as follows.

Bronchial tree: It consists of branches of bronchus, i.e. primary, secondary and terminal division of bronchus, lobular terminal and respiratory bronchioles:

- Bronchus and its branches are recognized by its characteristic four layers, i.e. mucosa, submucosa, cartilaginous layer and adventitia.
- Whereas bronchioles are the further subdivisions of the smaller bronchi, which consist of all the layers of bronchi with the lack of cartilaginous ring in it, terminal bronchioles are rich in a special type cells called **Clara cells.** Terminal and respiratory bronchioles are made up of a thin mucosal fold with lack of goblet cells in it. A small layer lamina propria and adventitia is also seen in association with it.

Alveolus: It is the **structural functional unit of lung,** which forms the end part of the bronchial tree:

a. An alveolus is a thin-walled polyhedral sac-like structure lined by simple squamous epithelium.
b. Here the epithelium is single layered, which rests on basement membrane. Deep to the basement membrane there is a delicate layer of loose areolar connective tissue through which numerous pulmonary capillaries run around. Epithelium lining the alveoli is called pneumocytes and a typical alveolus is lined by following types of epithelial cells (pneumocytes):
    - Types I cell: These are nothing, but the simple squamous epithelial cells with flat nucleus at the center and they form the major part of the alveolar cell population.
    - Types II cell: These are the modified simple squamous epithelial cells, which form about 8%–10% of total alveolar cells:
        - They bear fine microvilli on their surface with an abundant secretary granule in its cytoplasm.
    - Types III cells: These are very rare type cells with unknown functions. They are also called Brush cells.

Interalveolar septum: It is a thin layer of connective tissue found between the two alveoli. It is rich in numerous pulmonary capillaries, elastic fibers with a wide range of cells, which includes goblet cells, basal cells, mast cells, lymphocytes, serous cells, macrophages and Kulchitsky cells.

Functions

- Type I alveolar cell of lung tissue helps in exchange of respiratory gases between the alveoli of lung and pulmonary capillaries.

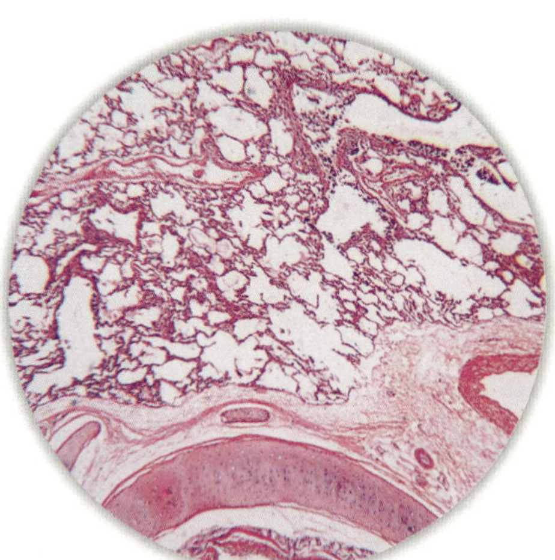

A

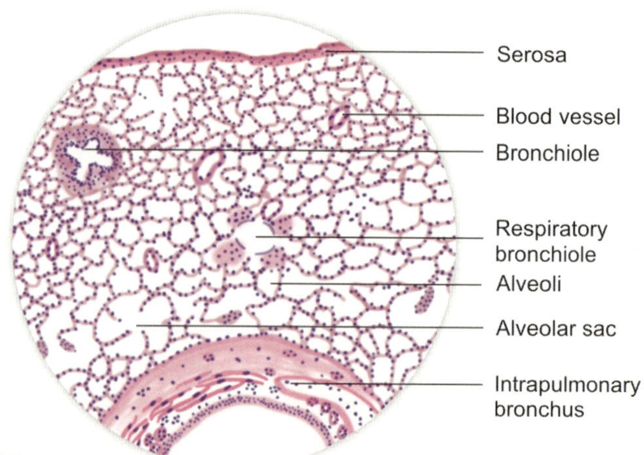

B

Figures 19.3A and B: Lung. **A.** Photograph; **B.** Diagrammatic representation.

- Types II alveolar cells including the cells of Clara secrete **surfactant,** which maintains the surface tension of the lung.
- **Kulchitsky cells** or **Feyrter cells** of lung belong to amine precursor uptake and decarboxylation (APUD) cell system and secrete some hormones and chemical substances like prostaglandins, serotonin, acetylcholine, etc.

Clinical Histology
Inflammation of the lung parenchyma is known as **pneumonia.**
Hyposecretion of surfactant in lung leads to **hyaline membrane disease** or **respiratory distress syndrome.**
In chronic **venous congestion of lung** minute capillaries become congested and rupture resulting in internal hemorrhage. Here hemosiderin released by red blood cells (RBCs) is taken by alveolar macrophages resulting in formation of **heart failure cells.**
Emphysema is a respiratory disorder caused due to the permanent dilatation of the air spaces with destruction of their walls.
Tuberculosis of the lung is most common and serious condition, which destroys the lung tissue and impairs its function.
Carcinoma of lung usually arises from type I alveolar epithelial cells.

- Mast cell present in the inter-alveolar septum secretes heparin thus prevents the intravascular blood clotting.
- Alveolar macrophages and lymphocytes act like second line of defense mechanism by engulfing the foreign bodies (dust, bacteria and other microorganisms).
- Regulation of acid-base balance, body temperature and water balance are also other functions of lung tissue.

Discussions

- How do you differentiate between bronchi and bronchioles microscopically?
- What is Clara cell and what is its function?
- Which is the structural and functional unit of lung?
- Name the different types of cells lining the alveolus and mention its functions.
- What is interlobular septum? What does it contain?
- What are Kulchitsky cells?
- Where do you see heart failure cells?
- What is pneumonia?
- What is emphysema?
- What is ARDS?

Chapter 20

Endocrine System

ENDOCRINE GLANDS

(Greek: Endo—inside; Krinein—to secrete)

- Endocrine glands are the type of glands, which produce hormones. Since they do not have ducts to carry their secretions, hence they are also called **ductless glands**.
- These glands are richly supplied by the blood vessels with fenestrated sinusoidal capillaries to carry their secretions.
- The endocrine system works closely in association with the nervous system, hence the expression **neuroendocrine system** is sometimes used.

HORMONE

(Greek: Hormaein—to set in motion)

- The word hormone comes from the Greek and was used for the first time in 1902 by two. British physiologists Starling and Bayliss.
- Hormone can be defined as **the chemical substances produced by the endocrine gland, which are required in minute quantity for the healthy growth and reproduction of an organism**.
- Hormones from the site of production, enter the bloodstream and act on the target organs to cause the changes in the activity of the target cells, hence they are also referred as **Chemical messengers**.

The important properties of hormones are:

- Hormones are secreted by the endocrine glands or tissues in small quantity, expressed in terms of nanograms per dL (ng/dL).
- They circulate in the blood to produce their effects, usually effects are seen on distant part of the body or not where they are produced.
- The effects are mostly seen on the target tissue or organ. The target tissue or organ may be another endocrine gland, exocrine gland or entirely different type of organ like bone, kidney, heart, etc.
- A single hormone can produce several effects on a single or several target tissues.
- The secretion of a hormone may depend upon another hormone or may be under the control of nervous system.
- The regulation of the hormone levels in the blood is either by negative feedback mechanism or positive feedback mechanism or both.
- All the hormones generally come under five different groups:
  - Steroids.
  - Amino acid derivatives.
  - Small peptides or proteins.
  - Glycoproteins.
  - Fatty acid derivatives.
- In general hypo- or hyper-secretion of any hormone leads to the change in the cellular activity of the target cell and endocrine glands, causing endocrine disorders.

The lists of important endocrine glands present in human body are as follows:

- Pineal gland
- Pituitary gland
- Thyroid gland
- Thymus
- Parathyroid glands
- Suprarenal glands
- Pancreas
- Testes (in male)
- Ovary (in female)
- Placenta (in pregnant female).

Note: Recent investigations have shown that liver also produces certain chemical substances called **somatomedins**, which are necessary for the growth of bones and other tissues or aids the functions of growth hormone.

Hence, liver is also considered as an endocrine organ, but it is still not universally accepted.

HYPOPHYSIS CEREBRI (PITUITARY GLAND)

Slide No. 49

Identification Points

- Pars anterior rich in cells and sinusoids
- Interglandular cleft with few colloidal vesicles
- Pars posterior with pituicytes and nerve fibers.

Introduction

- Pituitary gland (Figs 20.1A and B) is a small endocrine gland situated in the middle cranial fossa of the human skull.
- It is an oval-shaped gland measures about 8 mm anteroposteriorly and 12 mm transversely; it weighs about 500–600 mg.
- The gland is placed in a bony sac-like structure called **sella turcica**, which is a part of sphenoid bone.
- The gland is attached to the hypothalamus in the floor of the third ventricle by a stalk-like structure called **Infundibulum**.
- Pituitary gland is the chief gland, which controls the secretion of other endocrine glands either directly or indirectly; hence it is also called the master gland of endocrine system.

Development

- Embryologically, the anterior part of the pituitary develops from the Rathke's pouch as an upward projection of the buccopharyngeal epithelium, whereas the posterior pituitary develops from the base of the brain (hypothalamus) as a downward projection.
- Thus, anterior pituitary is ectodermal in origin and posterior pituitary is neuroectodermal in origin.

Subdivision of Hypophysis Cerebri (Figs 20.2 and 20.3)

- Pituitary gland is mainly divided into an anterior part called adenohypophysis and a posterior part called **neurohypophysis**.
- Adenohypophysis is further subdivided into pars anterior and pars intermedia. Pars anterior consists of two parts, i.e. pars tuberalis (tubular shaped) and pars distalis or glandularis (glandular part).
- The neurohypophysis consists of two parts, i.e. a posterior part called pars posterior and a tubular connecting part called infundibulum.
- The adenohypophysis of the gland has got rich vascular supply and also contains epithelial cells of varying sizes, they are arranged in cords or irregular follicles separated by sinusoids.

Chromophils and Chromophobes

The two important types of cells found in the adenohypophysis of the pituitary gland are:

- Chromophils: These constitute about 50% of the total cells in the adenohypophysis:

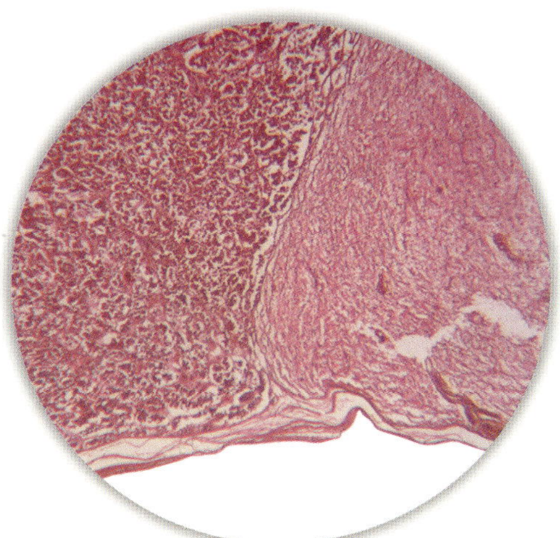

A

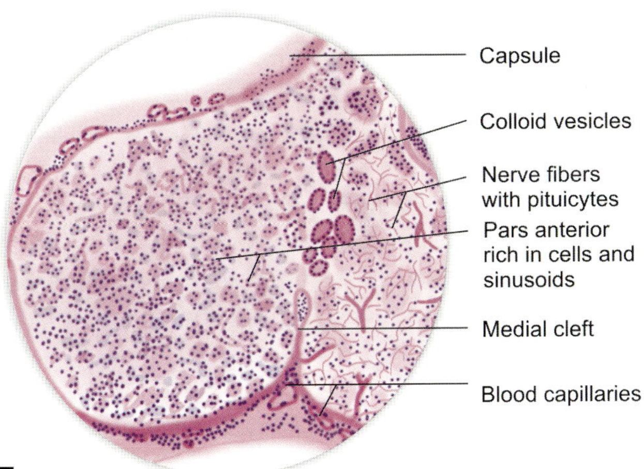

B

Figures 20.1A and B: Pituitary gland. **A.** Photograph; **B.** Diagrammatic representation.

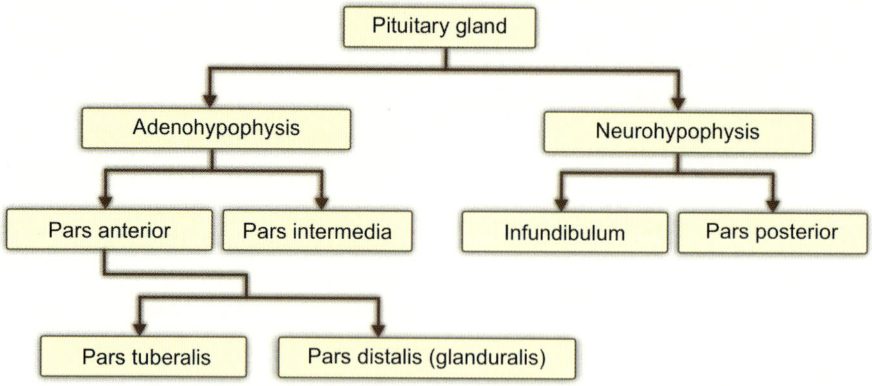

Figure 20.2: Subdivision of hypophysis cerebri

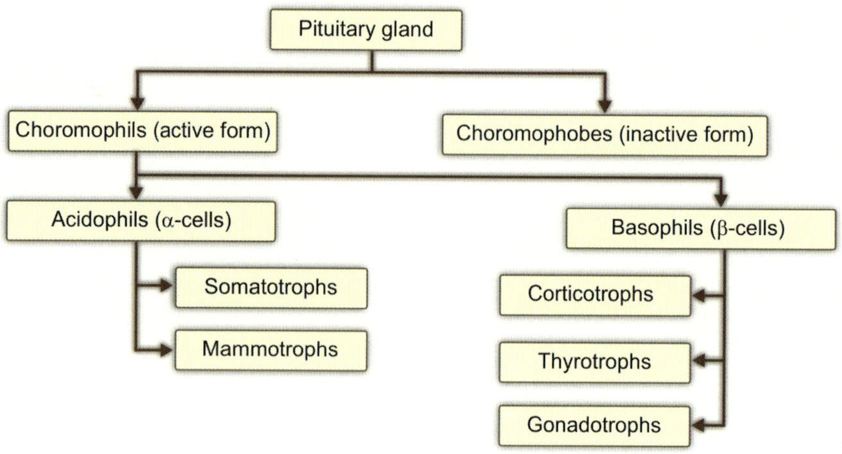

Figure 20.3: Cellular pattern of the hypophysis cerebri

- These are the cells having strong affinity for the staining dyes, have brightly stained granules in their cytoplasm.
- Chromophils are the active cells, which form the secretory part of the pituitary gland.

• Chromophobes: These constitute about rest of the 50% of the cells in the adenohypophysis:
  - These cells show less affinity for the staining dyes hence the granules are not properly stained or sometimes the cells will not be clear.
  - Chromophobes are the inactive part of the pituitary gland and these cells are rich in pars tuberalis of the adenohypophysis. On activation, chromophobe cells give rise to chromophil cells.

Chromophils are further classified into two types:

- Acidophils (α-cells): These are the type of chromophil cells having the affinity for dyes like eosin and orange G and they appear as pink-colored cells.
- Basophils (β-cells): These are the types of chromophil cells having the affinity for dyes like hematoxylin and they appear as purple to blue-colored cells. They are also stained by periodic acid-Schiff (PAS) method.

Based on the size and shape of the granules, both acidophils and basophils are further subdivided as given below.

Types of acidophils

Somatotrophs

Somatotrophs constitute about 50% of the total cells. They produce a hormone called somatotropin (STH) or growth hormone.

Actions of growth hormone

- Helps in the growth of almost all tissues of the body, which are capable of growing. It mainly increases the size and number of cells (hypertrophy and hyperplasia) by increasing the mitotic cell division.
- It also causes specific differentiation of the cells ike bone cells and muscle cells, etc.
- It acts on the bone cells and thus helps in increasing the length of the bone and its ossification.

In general, somatotrophic hormone is responsible for the normal growth of body, especially before puberty.

Mammotrophs or lactotrophs

Mammotrophs constitute about 25% of the total cells. They secrete a hormone called mammotrophic hormone (also called prolactin (PRL), lactogenic hormone).

Actions of mammotrophic hormone

- It increases the growth and activity of the mammary gland during pregnancy.
- It directly acts on epithelial cells of the mammary gland and causes localized alveolar hyperplasia, which is essential for milk production during lactation period.

Types of basophilic cells

Corticotrophs

Corticotrophs constitute about 15%–20% of the total cells populate. They secrete a hormone called corticotrophic hormone.

Actions of corticotrophic hormone

Stimulate the corticotrophic secretion of mineralocorticoids and glucocorticoids.

Thyrotrophs

Thyrotrophs are very few in number hardly constitute about 1%–5% of the total cells and they produce thyroid stimulating hormone (TSH).

Actions of TSH

- It stimulates the production of thyroxine and T3 in the thyroid gland.
- It controls the blood T3 and T4 level by negative feedback mechanism.
- It also controls the secretion of parafollicular cells of thyroid gland.

Gonadotrophs

They constitute about 10% of the total cell population. Gonadotrophs produce two types of hormones, i.e. follicle-stimulating hormone (FSH) and luteinizing hormone (LH).

Actions of FSH

In males: It stimulates the spermatogenesis in association with testosterone.

In females: It is responsible for the growth of the Graafian follicles and also causes the secretion of estrogen from the ovary.

Actions of LH

In males: It stimulates the interstitial cells of Leydig in testis to secrete testosterone hence, the hormone is also called **Interstitial cell stimulating hormone (ICSH)**.

In female

- It is responsible for the luteinization of ovum (release of ovum from ovary) hence called luteinizing hormone.
- It is also necessary for the formation of corpus luteum and secretion of progesterone hormone from the same.

Pars Intermedia and Pars Posterior

Pars intermedia:

Pars intermedia is a part of anterior pituitary where it is not well-developed in human beings, but very well-developed in lower animals:

- It is rich in follicles, which are lined by basophils and are believed to be the remnants of Rathke's pouch. It also contains few chromophobe cells.
- Functions of these cells are not clearly known. It is belived that they produce melanocyte stimulating hormone (MSH), ACTH and lipotropic hormone (LPH), but the predominant is MSH.
- The cells of pars intermedia belong to APUD cell system (APUD stands for amine precursor uptake decarboxylase).
- MSH acts on the melanocytes and causes pigmentation of skin thus giving brown to black color to the skin.

Pars posterior

- It is rich in unmyelinated nerve fibers, which are coming from the hypothalamus as a hypothalamohypophyseal tract; hence it is also called **pars nervosa**.
- This region is also rich in few dendritic cells called **pituicytes**.
- Pars posterior acts as storehouse of two hormones called antidiuretic hormone (ADH) and oxytocin.
- They are produced by the **supraoptic and paraventricular nuclei** of hypothalamus and the secretions from the hypothalamus are seen as small masses along the tract and are called **Herring bodies**.

Actions of ADH (vasopressin)

The ADH acts on the renal tubules of the nephron in kidney and helps in the absorption of water.

Actions of oxytocin

- It causes contraction of uterine muscles during the labor thus helps in the parturition of the baby.
- It also causes ejection of the milk from the mammary gland during lactation period.

Portal Circulation

- Since the pituitary gland is an important endocrine gland, to facilitate the vascularization and to carry the secretion of the gland, two sets of capillaries are arranged. This is called the portal system of the pituitary gland.
- Recent investigations have shown that even though the hormones are secreted by the adenohypophysis cells, initiations and regulation of their secretion is under the control of hypothalamus and it is mediated by neuroendocrine transducers.

Clinical Histology
Hyperpituitarism is a condition characterized by the over secretion of the pituitary hormones. For example: • Growth hormone—gigantism, acromegaly • ACTH—cushing's syndrome.
Hypopituitarism is a condition characterized by the less secretion of pituitary hormones. For example: • Growth hormones—dwarfism • ADH—diabetes insipidus.
Tumors of the pituitary gland may be seen in old age and usually tumors of the anterior pituitary are more common than the tumors of the posterior pituitary.

Discussions

- What is sella turcica?
- Why the pituitary gland is also called the master gland?
- What is infundibulum?
- Name the different parts of the pituitary gland.
- What is the development of pituitary gland?
- Name the hormones secreted by the following. What are their actions?
  - Anterior pituitary.
  - Pars intermedia.
  - Supraoptic.
  - Para ventricular nuclei.
- What are pituicytes?
- What are Herring bodies?
- What is portal system? Name two organs having portal system.
- What is another name for LH in men? Why is it called so?
- Which cells of the pituitary gland belong to APUD cell system?
- What is hypothalamohypophyseal tract?

THYROID GLAND

Slide No. 50

Identification Points

- Thyroid follicles lined by cuboidal epithelium
- Eosinophilic colloid in follicular cavity
- Parafollicular cells are seen.

Introduction

Thyroid gland (Figs 20.4A and B) is an endocrine gland situated in the lower part of the neck region and the gland lies against vertebrae C5, C6, C7 and T1:

- It is a butterfly-shaped gland, which consists of right and left lobes that are joined together by the isthmus.

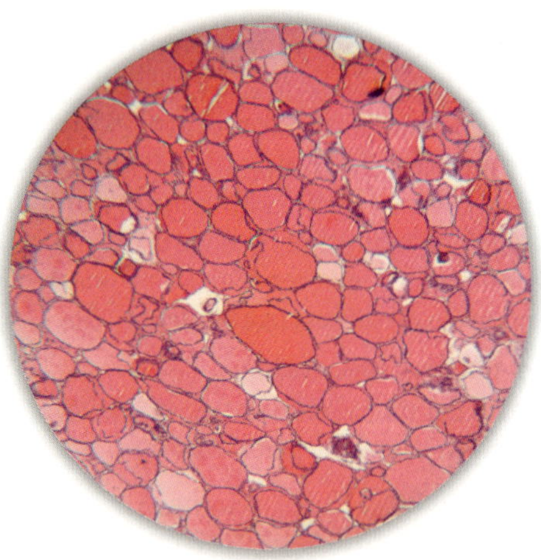

A

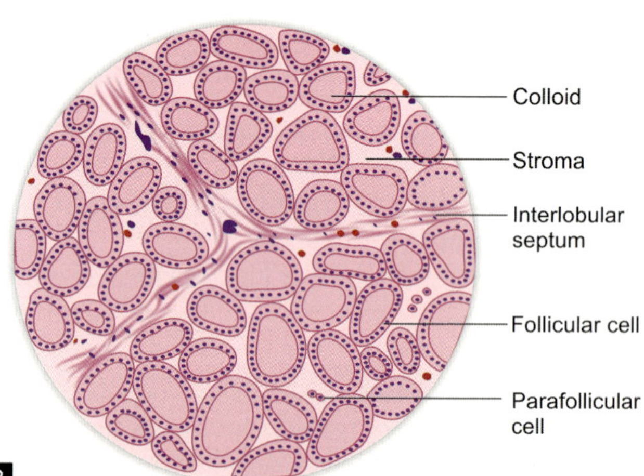

B

Figures 20.4A and B: Thyroid gland. **A.** Photograph; **B.** Diagrammatic representation.

- It is reddish brown in color and on average weighs about 25–30 g. The gland is known to be larger in females than males.
- It is covered by two capsules, i.e. an inner true capsule which is formed by the peripheral condensation by the connective tissue of the gland and an outer false capsule, which is derived from the pretracheal layer of the deep cervical fascia.
- The capsule enters the parenchyma of the gland forming connective tissue septa and thus divides the gland into many lobules.
- Thyroid gland is a unique gland among all the endocrine glands, as it can store large quantity of its hormonal secretions extracellularly; whereas most of the endocrine glands store their hormonal secretions intracellularly in small quantity.

Structure

Microscopically, thyroid gland is made up of two parts, i.e. the parenchyma and the stroma.

Stroma

- It is rich in loose areolar connective tissue with a delicate network of reticular fibers.
- It is seen in between the follicles of the gland; hence called **interfollicular connective tissue**.
- Stroma is rich in extensive network of lymphatic vessels, sympathetic nerve fibers, arterioles and capillaries, which are very close to the follicles of the gland.

Parenchyma

- Parenchyma of the gland is in the form of thyroid follicles.
- A follicle is a spherical shaped structure made up of follicular cells and are resting on the basement membrane.
- The follicle has a cavity, which is filled by a homogeneous, eosinophilic, material called **colloid**.
- Colloid is an iodized form of thyroglobulin, which is a glycoprotein chemically.
- It acts as the precursor form of T3 and T4 hormones and the amount of colloid present in the cavity depends upon the activity of the follicular cells.

Follicular cells

- Normally, these cells are cuboidal in shape, but the cell shape varies according to the activity of the cell.
- The cells are flat (squamous) in shape when they are inactive or in resting phase and the follicle is distended with a pool of colloid in it.
- The cells are cuboidal in shape when they are moderately active and the follicle is not distended with an adequate amount of colloid in it.
- The cells are columnar in shape when they are highly active or in secretory phase and there is scanty amount of colloid seen in the follicular cavity.
- Typically, a follicular cell shows microvilli on its surface and the cytoplasm is rich in rough endoplasmic reticulum and Golgi apparatus.
- They also contain lysosomes, microtubules and microfilaments.
- The apical part of the cell is rich in many secretory vacuoles. In addition to follicular cells, the parenchyma of the gland also contains another type of cells called **parafollicular cells**.

Parafollicular cells

- They are also called **clear cells or C cells or light cells**.
- These cells are polyhedral or oval with an eccentric nucleus, arranged singly or in groups.
- Typically, they are present in between the follicular cells and the basement membrane or may lie in the stroma of the gland.
- Parafollicular cell is also rich in rough endoplasmic reticulum, Golgi complex, mitochondria and membrane-bound secretory granules in it.
- The parafollicular cells belong to a special class of cell system called APUD cell system and they show **chromaffin reaction**.

Functions

- The follicular cells secrete two hormones called **thyroxine (T4) and triiodothyronine (T3)**, which play an important role in maintaining the basal metabolic rate and cellular metabolism (carbohydrate, protein and lipid).
- The parafollicular cells secrete a hormone called **calcitonin** and is helpful in reducing blood calcium level and its maintenance:
  - Decreased absorption of calcium in the gut.
  - Decreased bone resorption by osteoclasts.
  - Increased urinary excretion of calcium in the kidney.

Clinical Histology
Enlargement of the thyroid gland is known as **goiter**.
Hyperthyroidism is a condition where there is increased secretion of thyroid hormones in the body.
Hypothyroidism is a condition where there is decreased secretion of thyroid hormones in the body.
Inflammation of the thyroid gland is termed as **thyroiditis**.

Discussions

- What are the different forms of cells seen in the lining of thyroid follicle? What is their relation with the activity of the cell?
- What is the function of follicular cells?
- What are parafollicular cells? What do they secrete?
- What is a colloid?
- What is the relation between the colloid and the activity of the follicular cells?
- What is the location of parafollicular cells in the thyroid gland?
- What does stroma of the gland contain?
- What are the other names for the parafollicular cells?
- What are the actions of:
  - Thyroxine.
  - Calcitonin.

PARATHYROID GLAND

Slide No. 51

Identification Points

- Irregular cords of chief cells
- Large eosinophilic oxyphil cells
- Thyroid gland may be the accompanying structure.

Introduction

- Parathyroid glands (Figs 20.5A and B) are the two pairs of endocrine glands situated in the posterior border of the thyroid gland within the false capsule.
- Since they lie in close relationship to the thyroid gland; hence they are referred to as **parathyroid gland**.
- There are two parathyroid glands on each side of the neck called superior parathyroid gland and inferior parathyroid gland.
- Each parathyroid gland is an oval-shaped structure, yellowish brown in color, measuring 6 × 4 × 2 mm and weighs about 50 mg.

Development

- Embryologically, parathyroid gland develops in 4th to 5th week of intrauterine life.
- The superior parathyroid gland is derived from the fourth pharyngeal pouch whereas inferior parathyroid gland is derived from the third pharyngeal pouch of the primitive pharynges.

Structure

- Each gland is covered by a capsule, rich in dense irregular connective tissue.
- The septa of the connective tissue capsule enters the gland and thus divides it into irregular lobules.
- The microscopy of the parathyroid gland consists of two parts, i.e. stroma and parenchyma (Fig. 20.6).

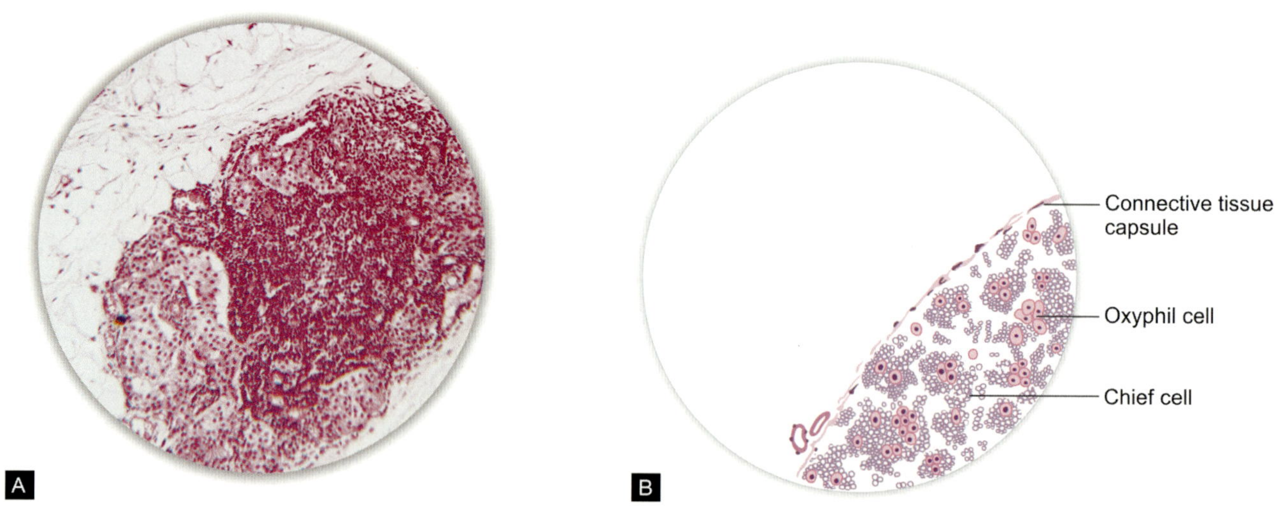

Figures 20.5A and B: Parathyroid gland. **A.** Photograph; **B.** Diagrammatic representation.

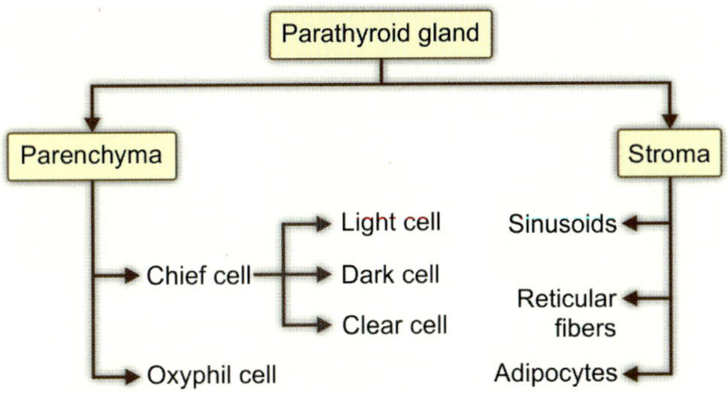

Figure 20.6: Classification of parathyroid gland

Stroma

- Stroma is rich in loose connective tissue with a delicate network of reticular fibers, which support the parenchyma of the gland. It is also rich in the blood capillaries and numerous sinusoids lying in close relation to the cells.
- As the age advances, the gland will be infiltrated by the adipocytes; hence many adipocytes are also seen in the stroma of the aged gland.

Parenchyma

Parenchyma is made up of wide, irregular, anastomosing cords of cells.

There are mainly two types of cells seen in the parenchyma:

a. **Chief cells:** It is also called **principal cell** and constitutes about 60%–70% of the total parenchyma.
   - It is a small, round- to oval-shaped cell with vesicular nucleus at the center with a homogeneous cytoplasm. It is also rich in rough endoplasmic reticulum and Golgi complex.
   - The chief cells are classified into three types based on its depth of their cytoplasmic staining and are:
     - Light cells
     - Dark cells
     - Clear cells.
   - Sometimes, these cells also contain glycogen and lipid in their cytoplasm.

b. **Oxyphil cell:** It is also called **eosinophil cells** and constitute about 30%–40% of the total parenchyma:
   - These cells appear just before the puberty and its number increases as the age advances.
   - An oxyphil is a large polygonal shaped cell with a dark, prominent small nucleus at the center. The cytoplasm contains highly eosinophilic granules in them, but the cells lack rough endoplasmic reticulum and Golgi complex.

Functions

- **Chief cell:** Chief cell is the main endocrine part of the gland and secretes a hormone called **parathormone (PTH)**, which increases the blood calcium level by:
  - Increased absorption of calcium from the gut.
  - Increased resorption of the bone (mobilization of calcium from bone).
  - Decreased excretion of calcium in the urine by kidney.
- **Oxyphil cells:** The exact function of the cell is not known and it does not secrete any hormones. However, it is proved that in pathological conditions, it may secrete parathormone.

Clinical Histology
Deficiency of parathormone causes **hypoparathyroidism**
Excess secretion of parathormone causes **hyperparathyroidism**

Discussions

- What is the location of parathyroid gland?
- What are the different types of cells seen in the parenchyma of the gland?
- What is the function of chief cell?
- What is the relation between the age of the gland and oxyphil cells?
- What is the function of oxyphil cell?
- Which cells of the parathyroid gland is rich in rough endoplasmic reticulum and Golgi apparatus?
- What is the action of parathormone?
- What is normal blood calcium level?
- Which organ is more important to the human body—thyroid gland or parathyroid gland?

SUPRARENAL GLAND (Supra—Above, Renal—Kidney)

Slide No. 52

Identification Points

- Outermost capsule with trabeculae
- Cortex showing zona glomerulosa, fasciculata and reticularis
- Medulla showing sinusoids and sympathetic ganglion cells.

Introduction

- Suprarenal glands (Figs 20.7A to C) are the pair of endocrine glands situated in the posterior abdominal wall above the upper pole of both the kidneys.
- As the name itself indicates, these are the pair of glands situated just above the kidney; hence called **suprarenal gland**.
- In many animals, they are found adjacent to the kidneys; hence they are also called **adrenal gland**.

Development

- Development of the suprarenal gland starts in the 5th week of fetal development.
- The medulla of the suprarenal gland is derived from the neural crest (ectoderm); whereas the cells of the cortex arise from the celomic epithelium (mesoderm) that lies in the angle between the developing gland and attachment of mesentery.

Structure

- The gland is enclosed by a thick layer of connective tissue capsule, which is rich in the collagen fibers.
- Many connective tissue septum arising from the capsule passes into the cortex. The gland is made up of two distinct functional parts:
  - Cortex.
  - Medulla.

Cortex

- It is the superficial outer part, which is 10 times wider than the medulla.

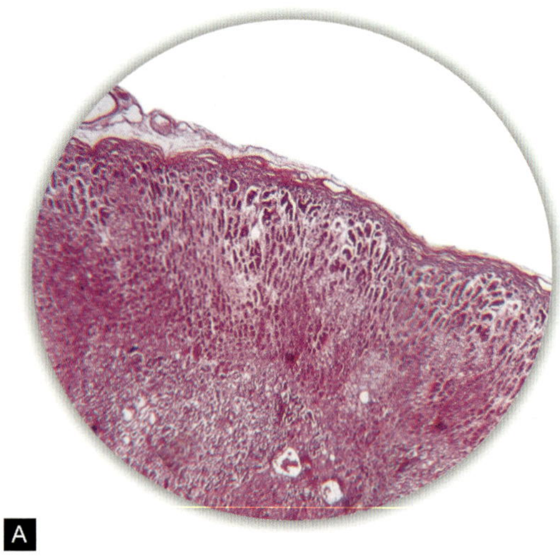

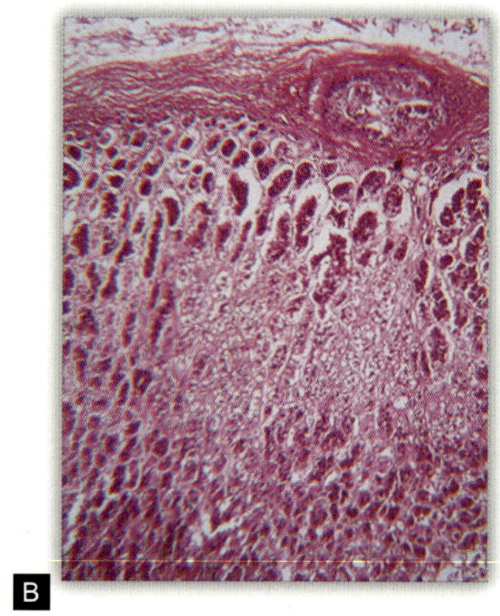

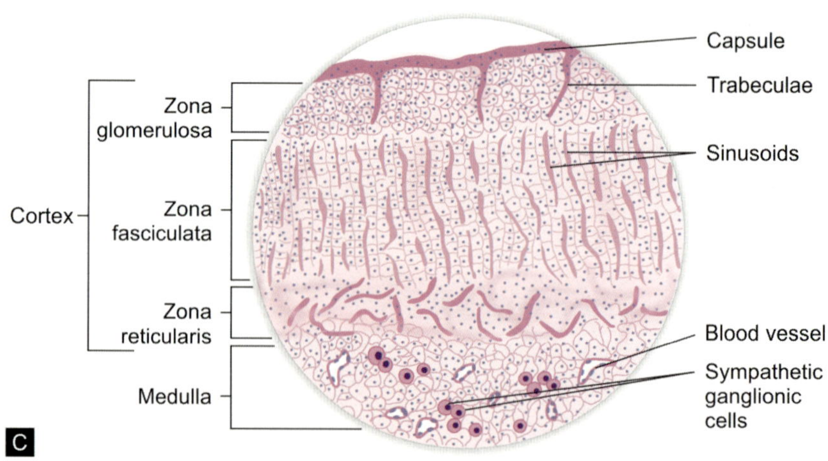

Figures 20.7A to C: Suprarenal gland. **A.** Photograph; **B.** Magnified view of capsule with cortex showing three different zones; **C.** Diagrammatic representation.

- It consists of three different layers of cells.
- From the periphery toward the center, these are named as:
  - Zona glomerulosa (one fifth of cortex).
  - Zona fasciculata (three fifth of cortex).
  - Zona reticularis (one fifth of cortex).

Zona glomerulosa

- It is the outermost layer of the cortex, which constitutes about one fifth of the total cortex. It is explained as follows:
  - **Cell shape:** Polyhedral or columnar.
  - **Arrangement:** Acinus-like groups or inverted 'U' form or horseshoe shaped.
  - **Cytoplasmic nature:** Basophilic.
- These cells contain prominent small nuclei with rich smooth endoplasmic reticulum and Golgi complex. Mitochondria are elongated in nature.

Functions

- The cells of zona glomerulosa secrete mineralocorticoids, e.g. aldosterone and 11-deoxycorticosterone.
- Mineralocorticoids are very essential in maintaining ionic concentration, electrolyte and water balance in the body.

Thus, aldosterone is also known as **life-saving hormone**.

Zona fasciculata

- It is the intermediate layer of the cortex which constitutes about 3/5th of the total cortex. It is explained as follows:
  - **Cell shape:** Polyhedral or columnar.
  - **Arrangement:** Cord like in two rows.
  - **Cytoplasmic nature:** Basophilic.
- These cells are also called **spongiocytes**; they contain large prominent nucleus with rich smooth endoplasmic reticulum. Golgi complex are best developed in the cells of zona fasciculata with spherical mitochondria.
- The cytoplasm of the cell is extensively vacuolated because of the presence of fat in it (can be demonstrated by Sudan dyes). These cells also store considerable amount of cholesterol and vitamin C.

Functions

- The cells of zona fasciculata secrete glucocorticoids with slight amount of mineralo-corticoids, e.g. corticosterone and cortisol (hydrocortisone).
- Glucocorticoids play an important role in the metabolism of carbohydrates, proteins and fats.
- Cortisol is known as **life-protecting hormone** since it helps to withstand the stress and trauma.
- The cells of zona fasciculata also secrete a small amount of **dehydroepiandrosterone (DHA)**.

Zona reticularis

- This is the innermost layer of the cortex which constitutes about one fifth of the total cortex. It is explained as follows:
  - **Cells shape:** Polyhedral or columnar.
  - **Arrangement:** Network like.
  - **Cytoplasmic nature:** Often acidophilic.
- These cells are more or less similar to that of zona fasciculata cells, but here the cords are branched to form a network-like structure. Hence, the name **zona reticulosa**.
- The cells are rich in smooth endoplasmic reticulum, Golgi apparatus, also contains small amount of fat in it. The mitochondria is unusual in shape with tubular cisternae. Few cells of zona reticularis often contain brown pigment.

Functions

- The cells of zona reticularis secrete predominantly sex hormones with small amount of glucocorticoids.
- These sex hormones induce the secondary sexual haracters in both males (androgen) and females (estrogen).

Medulla

- Medulla is the innermost part of the suprarenal gland, which constitutes about one tenth of the total gland. It is explained as follows:
  - **Cell shape:** Polyhedral or columnar.
  - **Arrangement:** Clumps and irregular cords with sinusoids.
  - **Cytoplasmic nature:** Basophilic.
- The cells of medulla are considered as the modified postganglionic sympathetic neurons.
- These cells are rich in secretory granules with abundant rough endoplasmic reticulum and Golgi complex.

Chromaffin reaction: When a sample of tissue is fixed in a solution containing the salts of chromium, (chromium sulfate, potassium dichromate, etc.) the cells show yellow-colored granules in their cytoplasm.

Such cells are called chromaffin cells and the process is known as **chromaffin reaction**, and the cells of the adrenal medulla belong to chromaffin cell system.

Functions

Cells of the adrenal medulla secrete catecholamines, which include:

- Adrenaline (epinephrine)
- Noradrenaline (norepinephrine)
- Dopamine.

Clinical Histology
Hypersecretion of glucocorticoid causes **Cushing's syndrome**.
Hyposecretion of corticosteroid causes **Addison's disease**.
Pheochromocytoma is a condition resulting due to excess secretion of catecholamines from medulla.

They act as neurotransmitters and also play an important role in cardiac function and maintenance of normal blood pressure.

Discussions

- What is suprarenal gland? Why is it called so?
- What is the development of suprarenal gland?
- Which are the different layers of cortex?
- Name the hormones secreted by:
  - Zona glomerulosa.
  - Zona fasciculata.
  - Zona reticularis.
  - Medulla.
- Which layer of the cortex is rich in cells containing fat vacuoles and vitamin C?
- Which hormone is referred to as:
  - Life-saving hormone.
  - Life-protecting hormone.
- What are spongiocytes?
- What is chromaffin reaction?
- Name few cells showing chromaffin reaction?
- Which part of the suprarenal gland is important for the life and why?

Chapter 21 Male Reproductive System

INTRODUCTION

- Male reproductive system consists of a pair of testis, epididymis, vas deferens, seminal vesicles, prostate, bulbourethral glands and penis (Fig. 21.1).
- Testis is the main sex organ responsible for the production of sperms. Hence, it is considered as **primary sex organ** and rest of the parts are said to be **accessory sex organs.**
- Penis is common for both renal system and male reproductive system and here it is the organ of copulation.

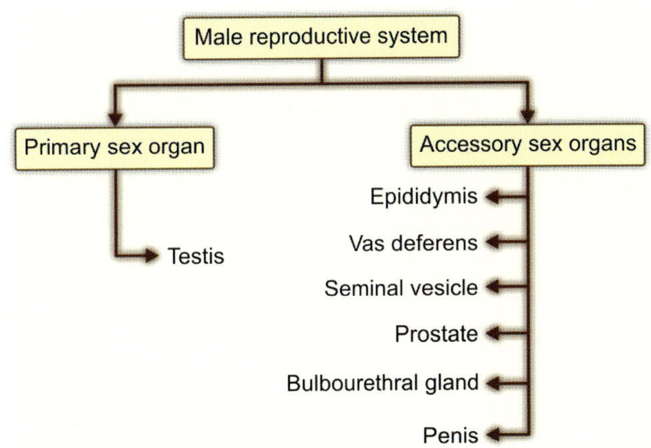

Figure 21.1: Male reproductive system

TESTIS

Slide No. 53

Identification Points

- Numerous seminiferous tubules
- Interstitial cells of Leydig present
- Sertoli cells in seminiferous epithelium.

Introduction

- Testis (Figs 21.2A and B) is a pair of male reproductive organ placed in a sac-like structure called scrotum.

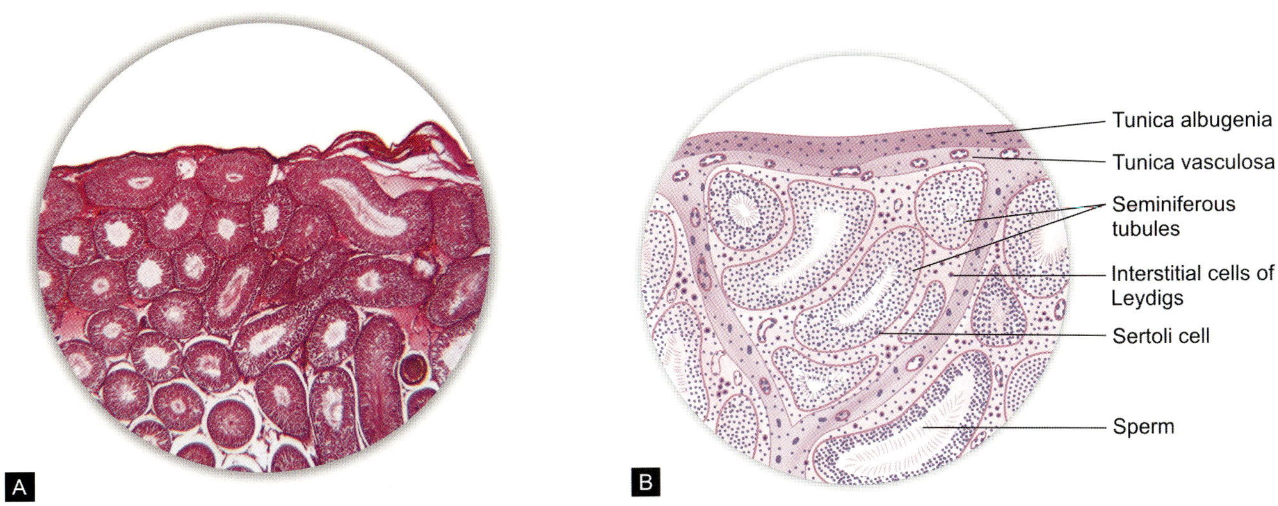

Figures 21.2A and B: Testis. **A.** Photograph; **B.** Diagrammatic representation.

- A typical testis is an oval-shaped structure surrounded by a serous sac, derived from peritoneum called Tunica vaginalis.

Structure

A detailed structure of transverse section (TS) of testis is explained as follows.

Tunica albuginea: It is an outermost layer of thick dense irregular connective tissue rich in collagen fibers and few elastic fibers:

- In posterior part of testis it expands and projects into the substance of testis as **mediastinum testis**.

Tunica vasculosa: It is internal layers of loose connective tissue rich in blood capillaries hence the name given **Tunica vasculosa**:

- The connective tissue of mediastinum testis extends into the testis as thin septae and divide the whole testis into numerous lobules.

Testicular lobule: There are about 200 testicular lobules in testis and each lobule contains one to four seminiferous tubules in it.

Seminiferous tubule: It is a coiled tubular structure present in the testicular lobules (Figs 21.3A and B):

- On an average each testis contains about 600 seminiferous tubules in it.
- Internally, a seminiferous tubule is lined by stratified germinal epithelium also known as **seminiferous epithelium**.
- Seminiferous epithelium consists of two distinct type of cells and are proliferative **spermatogenic cells** and non-proliferative **Sertoli cells** (Fig. 21.4).

Spermatogenic cells: These are germ cells of seminiferous tubules, which undergo a series of growth, multiplication and differentiation phase finally forming an active sperms and the phenomenon is known as spermatogenesis.

Sertoli cells: These are the non-proliferative forms of cells also called **sustentacular cells**.

- Typically, they are tall, slender and an irregular columnar-shaped cells with a large prominent nucleus at its base.
- Here, the base of the cell always rests on basement membrane and the apex bears many complicated recesses into which spermatid and sperms are fitted.

Functions

- It nourishes spermatogonial cells.
- It supports spermatogonial cells.
- Phagocytic in nature hence acts as macrophage.
- Secretes prostaglandins
- Secretes a hormone called **inhibin,** which inhibits the release of FSH from anterior pituitary.

The space between seminiferous tubules is filled by loose areolar connective tissue containing blood vessels and modified epithelial cells called **interstitial cells of Leydig**.

Interstitial cells of Leydig: It is a modified epitheliocyte seen in interstitial space as clusters of cells.

- The cytoplasm of cell contains yellow pigment granules in it and they are said to belong to APUD cell system (APUD stands for 'amine precursor uptake decarboxylase').

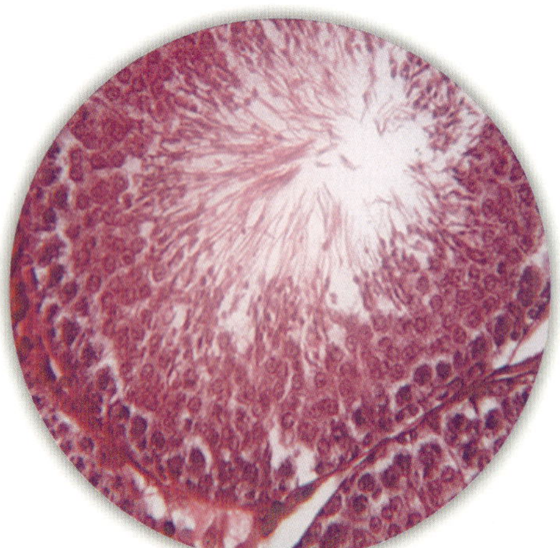

A

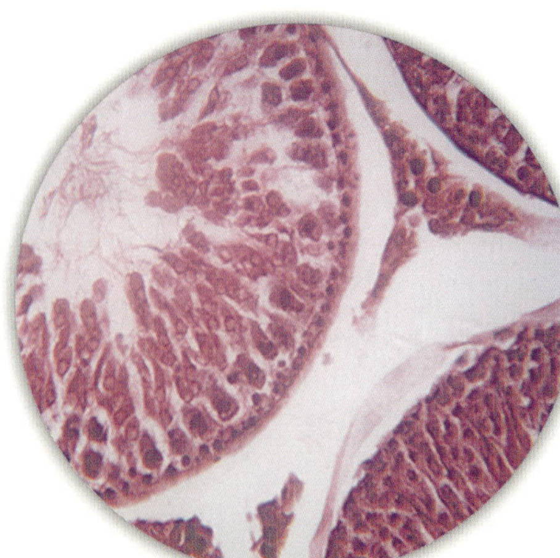

B

Figures 21.3A and B: Seminiferous tubules (with interstitial cells of Leydig)

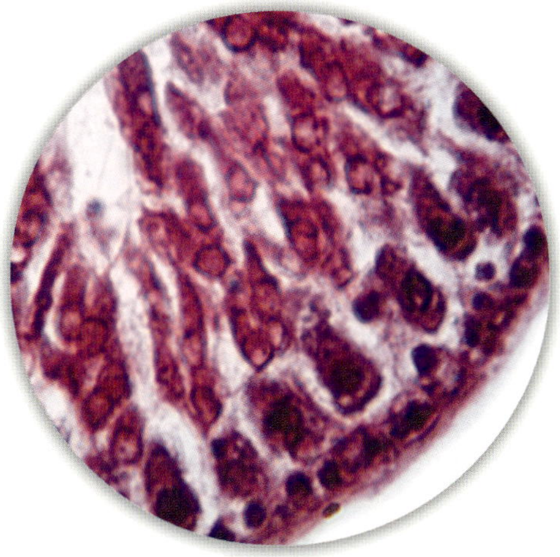

Figure 21.4: Seminiferous tubule showing spermatogenic cells and Sertoli cells

Function

Interstitial cells of Leydig produce a male sex hormone called **testosterone,** which is essential for the appearance of secondary sexual characters in male.

Discussions

- Name the coverings of testis.
- What are testicular lobules? What do they contain?
- Name the internal lining of seminiferous tubules.
- What are spermatogonial cells? What are their functions?
- What are Sertoli cells? List their functions.
- What is spermiogenesis and spermatogenesis?
- What are interstitial cells of Leydig? What do they do?
- Name a syndrome associated with hypogonadism in males.

Clinical Histology
The process of spermatogenesis requires 1°C–2°C less than body temperature. That is why the testes are placed outside the body in scrotum: • Failure of embryonic descent of testis leads to sterility in men and is known as **cryptorchidism**
Hyposecretion of gonadotropic hormone leads to testicular atrophy, which manifests as **enuchism**
Frolich's syndrome and Klinefelter's syndrome are the two important syndromes characterized by the hypogonadism in adolescent men

EPIDIDYMIS (TS)

Slide No. 54

Identification Points

- Tubules lined by pseudostratified columnar epithelium
- Sperms in the tubular lumen
- Thin circular muscle layer surrounding the ducts.

Introduction

- Epididymis is a coiled tube-like structure present on posterolateral aspect of testis (Figs 21.5A and B).
- Morphologically, it is divided into head, body and tail where head is the continuation of efferent ductules whereas body and tail is made up of canal of epididymis.

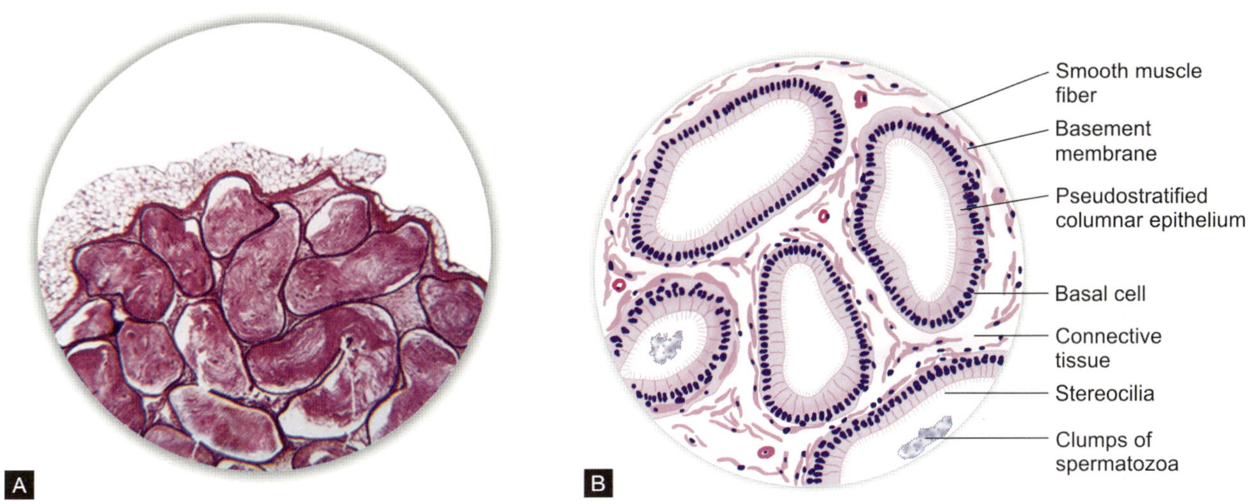

Figures 21.5A and B: Epididymis [transverse section (TS)]. **A.** Photograph; **B.** Diagrammatic representation.

Structure

- A transverse section (TS) of epididymis shows sections of canal of **ductus epididymis** lined by pseudostratified columnar epithelium and basal cells.
- Pseudostratified columnar epithelium is the principal cell with a tall columnar shape.
- They bear multinuclei at its base of cell, whereas apex bears numerous non-motile projections (microvilli) that resemble cilia and are called **stereocilia**.

Functions

- Phagocytosis of defective sperms.
- Concentration of semen by water absorption from it.
- Secretes glycoproteins (sialic acid, glycerylphosphorylcholine), which is essential for maturation of spermatozoas.

Basal cells: These are the small rounded or polyhedral cells found in between the bases of tall columnar principle cells.

Functions

- Basal cells are believed to be the stem cells, which give rise to pseudostratified columnar cells.

  In between the ductus epididymis, there is a loose areolar connective tissue with circular smooth muscles surrounding the tubules. Contraction of these muscles leads to expulsion of sperms from lumen of epididymis.

Discussions

- Name the different parts of epididymis.
- What is ductus epididymis?
- Name the internal lining of ductus epididymis.
- What are principal cells? What are their functions?
- What are basal cells? Where do you find them?
- What do you see in the lumen of ductus epididymis?
- What is the role of smooth muscle fibers surrounding the ductus epididymis?
- What is stereocilia?

VAS DEFERENS (TS)

Slide No. 55

Identification Points

- Small stellate lumen
- Lined by pseudostratified ciliated columnar epithelium
- Thick muscle coat of inner longitudinal, middle circular and outer longitudinal layer.

Introduction

Ductus (vas) deferens is a long elongated tube-like structure, originates as continuation of tail of epididymis. Its terminal (distal) part expands to form **ampulla,** which opens into ejaculatory duct after joining seminal vesicles (Figs 21.6A and B).

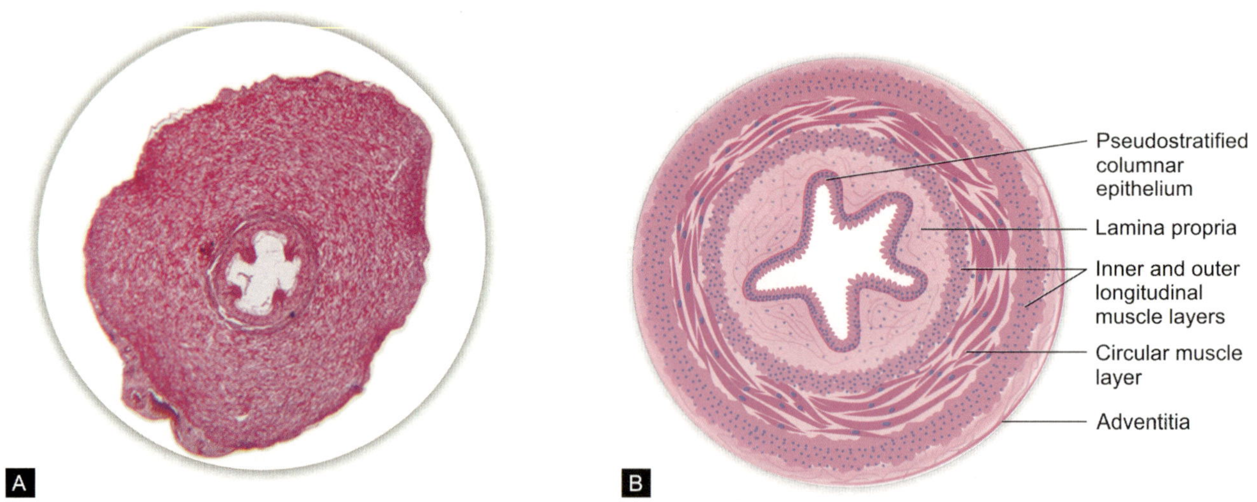

Figures 21.6A and B: Vas deferens [transverse section (TS)]. **A.** Photograph; **B.** Diagrammatic representation.

Structure

A typical TS of vas deferens shows the following three layers.

Mucosa: It is the innermost layer of vas deferens lined by pseudostratified columnar epithelium (Fig. 21.7):

- Here, the nucleus of cell is situated at its base whereas the apex bears numerous stereocilia on it. And here all the cells are resting on basement membrane.
- Underneath the basement membrane, there exists lamina propria containing compactly arranged collagen fibers with few elastic fibers in it.
- Mucosa of vas deferens is thrown into many longitudinal folds, which gives a **stellate shape**.

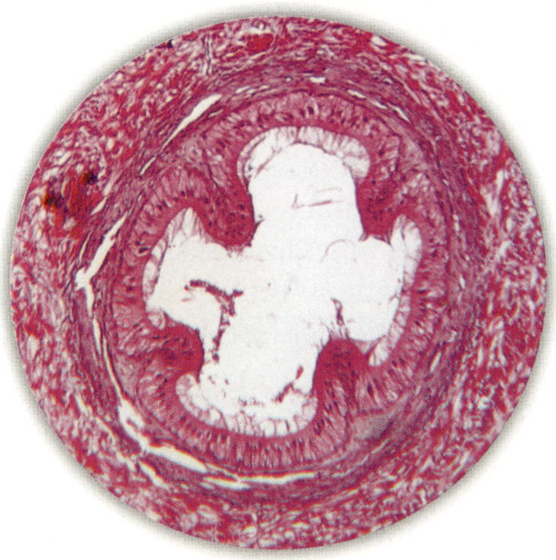

Figure 21.7: Note the lumen and pseudostratified ciliated columnar epithelium lining the vas deferens

Muscular layer: This in vas deferens is very prominent and consists of inner longitudinal, middle circular and outer longitudinal muscle coat.

Adventitia: It is the outermost layer made up of dense irregular connective tissue with blood vessels and nerve fibers embedded in it.

Functions

- Pseudostratified columnar epithelium lining the mucosa is both secretory and absorptive in function.
- Powerful contractions of muscle coat make sperms to move toward the ejaculatory duct.
- Adventitial layer is protective and supportive in function.

Discussions

- What is ampulla?
- Name the layers of vas deferens.
- Name the epithelium lining the mucosa of vas deferens.
- Enumerate the mode of arrangement of smooth muscles in vas deferens.
- Which is the outermost layer of vas deferens? What is it made up of?

SEMINAL VESICLE (TS)

Slide No. 56

Identification Points

- Branching and anastomosing mucosal folds
- Mucosa lined by pseudostratified columnar epithelium
- Muscular coat of inner circular muscle and outer longitudinal muscles.

Introduction

- Seminal vesicles are the pair of accessory sex organs situated on posterior side of urinary bladder (Figs 21.8A and B).
- It is an elongated sac-like structure, which opens into ejaculatory duct.

Structure

Mucosa: It is the innermost layer of seminal vesicle made up of complicated mucosal folds, which branches and anastomoses each other giving rise to **honeycomb appearance**:

- Epithelial lining of mucosa is highly variable. Generally, it is said to be low pseudostratified columnar, but at some places, it could be low columnar or cuboidal also.
- Here, the cellular pattern varies with extent of secretary activities.
- Just below the epithelium there is a lamina propria rich in elastic fibers, which forms the core of larger primary folds of mucosa.

Muscular layer: Here, it is not prominent as that of vas deferens and is made up of inner circular and outer longitudinal muscle layer.

Adventitia: Found beneath the muscular layer made up of dense connective tissue containing few blood vessels in it.

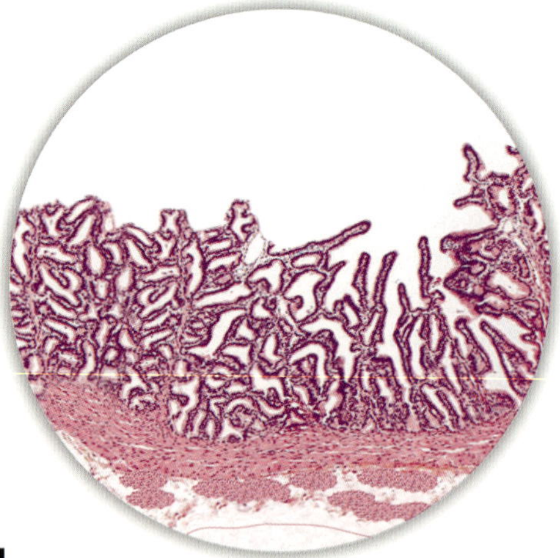

A

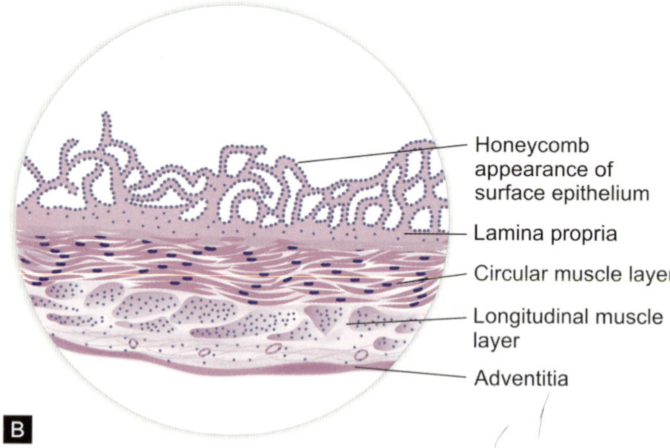

B

Figures 21.8A and B: Seminal vesicle [transverse section (TS)]. **A.** Photograph; **B.** Diagrammatic representation.

Functions

- Epithelium lining the mucosa is secretary in function and they secrete a semisolid, viscous fluid called **semen**. Semen is an alkaline fluid rich in glucosaminoglycans and fructose, which nourishes the spermatozoas.
- Muscular layer helps in ejaculation of semen into ejaculatory duct.
- Adventitia is protective and supportive in function.

Discussions

- List the different layers of seminal vesicle.
- What is the special feature of mucosa of seminal vesicle?
- What are the differences between muscular layer of vas deferens and of seminal vesicle?
- Which is the outermost layer of seminal vesicle?
- Enumerate the functions of seminal vesicle.
- What is semen? What does it contain?

PROSTATE

Slide No. 57

Identification Points

- Prostatic acini are lined by simple columnar epithelium
- Fibromuscular stroma
- Corpora amylacea in the lumen.

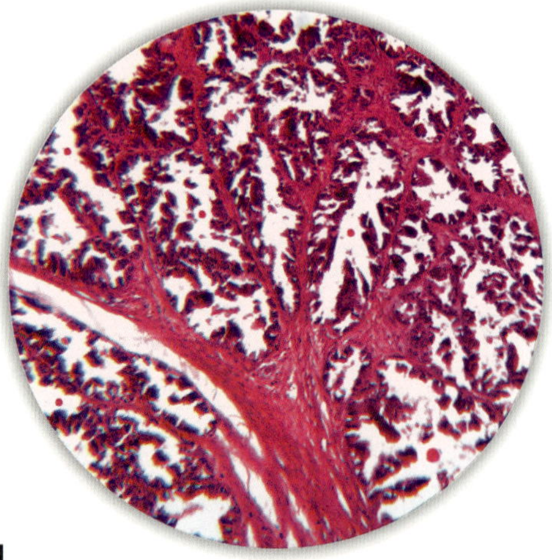

A

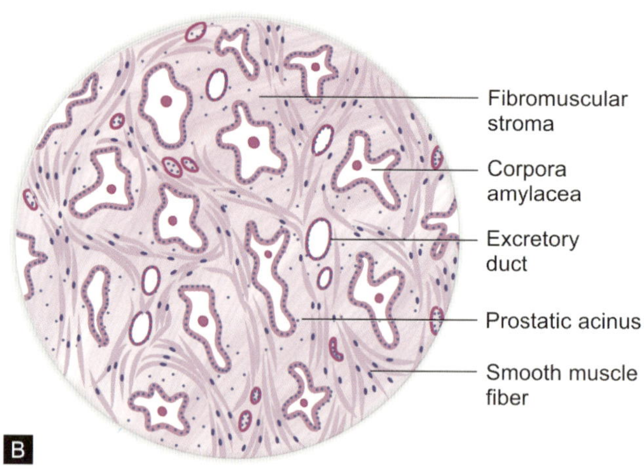

B

Figures 21.9A and B: Prostate. **A.** Photograph; **B.** Diagrammatic representation.

Introduction

- Prostatic gland is an accessory male sex organ found inferior to the neck of urinary bladder (Figs 21.9A and B).
- It is a **fibromusculoglandular structure** made up of **compound tubuloalveolar gland**.

Structure

A detailed structure of prostate can be explained under the following headings.

Capsule: It has an inner **true capsule** formed by the condensation of fibromuscular stroma and an outer **false capsule** made up of pelvic fascia. In between the two capsule layers there is a rich venous plexus network.

Parenchyma: The parenchyma of prostate is made up of 300–500 compound tubuloalveolar glands.

- Each gland is lined by simple columnar epithelium resting on basement membrane.
- Here, the size of gland is highly variable with an irregularity in its lumen shape.
- Some prostatic glands contain solid secretory aggregations, which appear as amorphous, eosinophilic bodies and are called **amyloid body** or **corpora amylacea**.
- The exact function of corpora amylacea is not known. Since, they appear as the age advances hence it has a medicolegal importance in estimating the age of an individual.
- An amyloid body is formed by the condensation of glycoprotein secreted by the columnar epithelium, which usually calcifies as the time passes.

Stroma: This of the gland is said to be peculiar as it is made up of both fibrous elements and muscular elements:

- Fibrous elements include numerous collagen fibers with fibroblasts in it and bundles of muscle fibers form the muscular elements.
- Apart from this fibromuscular stroma, it is also rich in blood vessels with few excretory ducts of prostatic glands lined by columnar cells.

Functions

- Simple columnar epithelium lining the prostatic gland secretes a thin, milky alkaline fluid which forms 30% of total semen. This secretion is rich in sodium salts, cholesterol, phospholipids, spermine, fibrinolysin and few clotting enzymes.
- Prostate is also said to secrete a hormone called **prostaglandin**.

Clinical Histology
Benign prostatic hypertrophy is a physiological condition occurring after the age of 50, which manifests as urinary incontinence due to the hypertrophy of prostatic glands
Malignant transformation of prostatic gland results in **carcinoma of prostate**

Discussions

- Describe the capsule of prostate gland.
- Name the epithelium lining the prostatic glands.
- What are corpora amylacea? What is its significance?
- Why is the stroma of prostate peculiar?
- List the functions of prostate gland.
- What is benign prostatic hypertrophy?

CHAPTER

22

Female Reproductive System

INTRODUCTION

- Female reproductive system (Fig. 22.1) consists of external and internal sex organs.
- Internal sex organs include a pair of ovary, a pair of fallopian tube, uterus and vagina, whereas external genitalia and mammary glands are considered as external genital organs.

OVARY

Slide No. 58

Identification Points

- Tunica albuginea with germinal epithelium
- Cortex showing ovarian follicles of different stages
- Medulla showing blood vessels.

Introduction

- Ovary (Figs 22.2A and B) is a pair of female reproductive organ situated in the ovarian fossa of pelvic cavity.
- It is an almond-shaped structure situated very close to fimbriae and are held in position by ovarian ligament and broad ligament by a fold of peritoneum, the mesovarium.

Structure

Germinal epithelium: It is an outermost layer of ovary lined by single layer of simple cuboidal epithelium:

- An outer surface of germinal epithelium is continuous with the mesothelium of visceral peritoneum and inner surface of germinal epithelium rests on a layer of dense irregular connective tissue called **tunica albuginea.**

  Note: The term 'germinal epithelium' is a misnomer here, as unlike the germinal epithelium of testis, it does not produce any germ cells.
- The tunica albuginea of ovary is much thinner and less dense than that of tunica albuginea of testis.

Cortex: It forms the major part of ovary and lies just below the tunica albuginea.

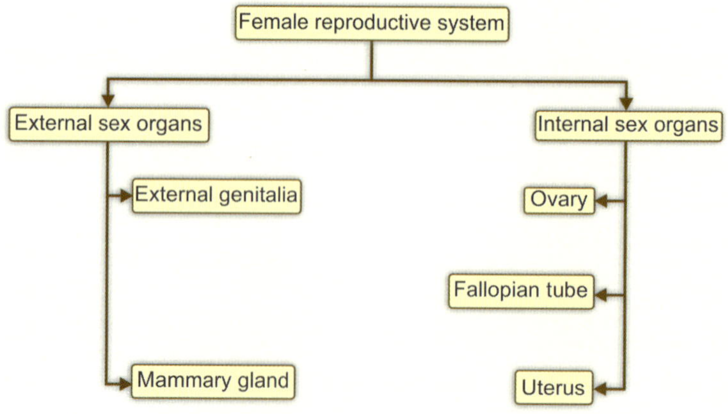

Figure 22.1: Female reproductive system

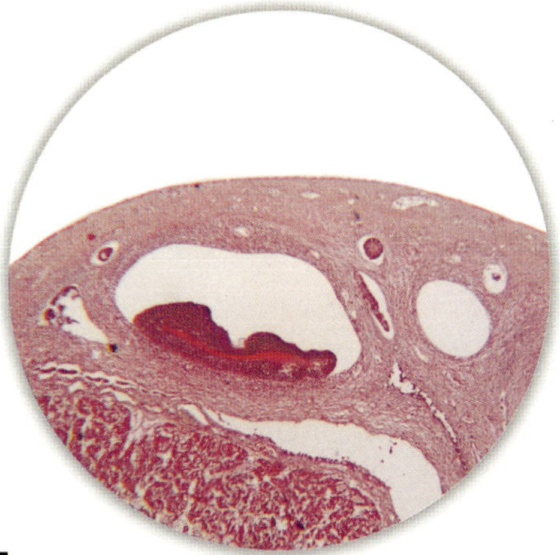

A

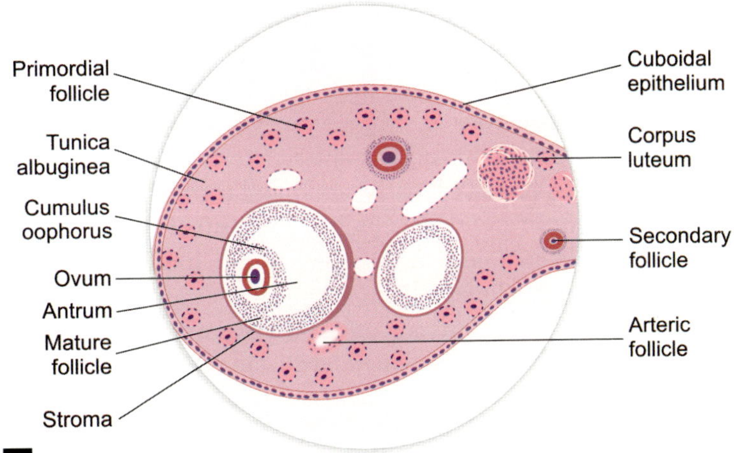

B

Figures 22.2A and B: Ovary. **A.** Photograph; **B.** Diagrammatic representation.

Stroma of ovarian cortex is made up of an extensive network of reticular fibers, few collagen fibers with a spindle-shaped fibroblasts called **fusiform cells.** Stroma is filled with numerous ovarian follicles of different stages and they are:

- Primordial follicle
- Primary follicle
- Secondary follicle
- Tertiary follicle
- Corpus luteum.

a. **Primordial follicle:** These are the most numerous follicles located in the periphery of the ovarian cortex:
   - They are the smallest and simplest structures made up of a primary oocyte and a single layer of squamous follicular cells surrounding it.

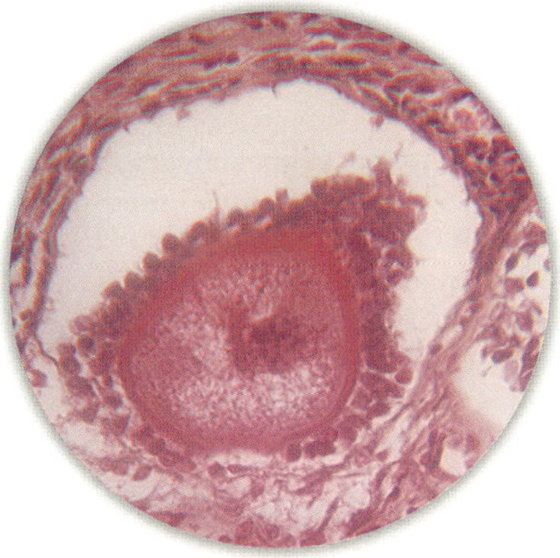

Figure 22.3: Graafian follicle showing ovum with zona pellucida and cumulus oophorus

a. **Primary follicle:** It is a modified primordial follicle with following growth:
   - Primary oocyte increases in size
   - Flattened squamous follicular cells become multilayered and rest on a thick basement membrane
   - A layer of glycoprotein, i.e. **zona pellucida** separates primary oocyte from the follicular cells
   - Stroma of the ovarian cortex surrounding the primary follicle forms theca folliculi.

c. **Secondary follicle:** It is also called **antral follicle,** since, it contains a crescentic space called **antrum.** Salient features of secondary follicle are:
   - Oocytes increase in size
   - Formation of antrum with liquor of folliculi
   - Theca folliculi are differentiated into inner theca interna and outer theca externa.

d. **Tertiary follicle:** It is the largest mature follicle of ovarian cortex also called **graafian follicle.** A typical mature graafian follicle (Fig. 22.3) shows following features:
   - Contains primary oocyte surrounded by zona pellucida
   - Primary oocyte is protected by a single layer of granulosa cells forming corona radiata, which in turn, is surrounded by a huge mass of cells called **cumulus oophorus**
   - Large antrum containing liquor of folliculi, protruded by cumulus oophorus
   - A multilayered cells lining the wall of antrum forming **membrane granulosa**
   - An inner theca interna rich in blood vessels and estrogen secreting glands, surrounded by an outer theca externa made up of fibrous connective tissue.

e. **Corpus luteum:** It is formed after ovulation stage from the ovulated (ruptured) graafian follicle. A corpus luteum is:
   - Collapsed, highly folded and modified temporary endocrine gland.
   - Membrana granulosa cells enlarge in size with an accumulation of yellowish carotenoid pigment in it called **lutein** and such cells are called **luteal cells.**
   - Theca internal cells also undergo same modification adding cellular bulk.
   - Corpus luteum starts secreting progesterone with a small amount of estrogen, if fertilization has taken place. If not it turns into a degenerating form called **corpus albicans.**

Medulla: It is made up of connective tissue rich in blood vessels, elastic fibers and few smooth muscles also.

Functions

Before ovulation: Thecal glands present in theca interna of graafian follicle secretes estrogen hormone, which is responsible for the appearance of secondary sexual characters in females.

After ovulation: Luteal cells of the corpus luteum secretes progesterone hormone and a small amount of estrogen, which maintains the pregnancy, if the fertilization has taken place.

Discussion

- What is germinal epithelium? What are the differences between germinal epithelium of ovary and that of testis?
- What is tunica albuginea? What are the differences between tunica albuginea of ovary and that of tests?
- Which stage of follicles are numerous in the ovarian cortex?
- List the different stages of ovarian follicles and mention few significant changes of each stage.
- Explain the structure of a mature graafian follicle in detail.
- What is cumulus oophorus? What does it contain?
- Explain the following terms:
  - Zona pellucida.
  - Corona radiata.
  - Antrum.
  - Theca folliculi.
  - Corpus luteum.
  - Corpus albicans.
  - Arteric follicle.
- What is ovulation?
- Which hormone regulates the development of ovarian follicles?

FALLOPIAN TUBE

Slide No. 59

Identification Points

- Highly folded mucosa
- Mucosa lined by simple columnar (ciliated) epithelium
- Inner circular and outer longitudinal muscle coat.

Introduction

- Fallopian tube (uterine tube) is a hollow tubular structure (Figs 22.4A and B), which conveys the oocyte from ovary to uterus.
- The different parts of fallopian tube are isthmus, ampulla and infundibulum.
- It is made up of inner mucosa, middle muscular coat with an outer serosa.

Mucosa: It is predominantly lined by simple columnar epithelium, resting on basement membrane. However, ciliated columnar epithelium along with few intercalary cells are also present in lining the surface epithelium:

- Mucosa of the fallopian tube is thrown into numerous branching folds, which fill the whole lumen.
- Mucosal folds are filled with loose connective tissue forming lamina propria.

Muscular coat: It is seen just below the lamina propria and made up of inner circular and outer longitudinal muscle fibers with an abundant interstitial connective tissue.

Serosa: It is the outermost layer consisting of mesothelium of peritoneum with few connective tissue components.

Functions

- The ciliated columnar epithelium helps in movement of sperms and ovum towards each other, thus facilitating the fertilization.
- Simple columnar epithelial cells are secretory in nature and their secretion is responsible for the nourishment of fertilized ovum till its implantation.
- Contraction of muscle fibers of muscular coat also aids the process of fertilization.

Discussion

- Name the different layers in fallopian tube.
- Describe the mucosa of fallopian tube.

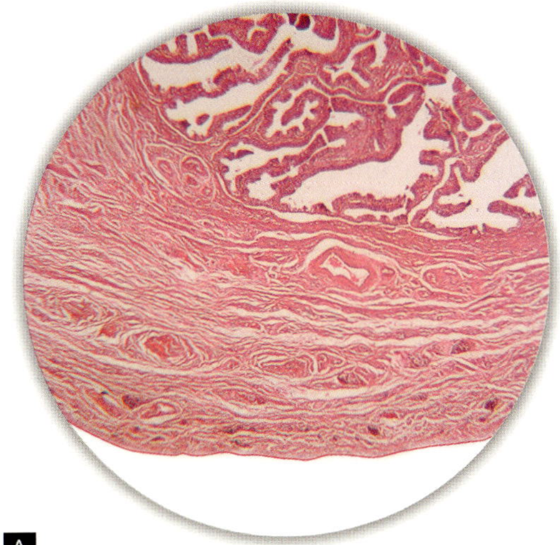

A

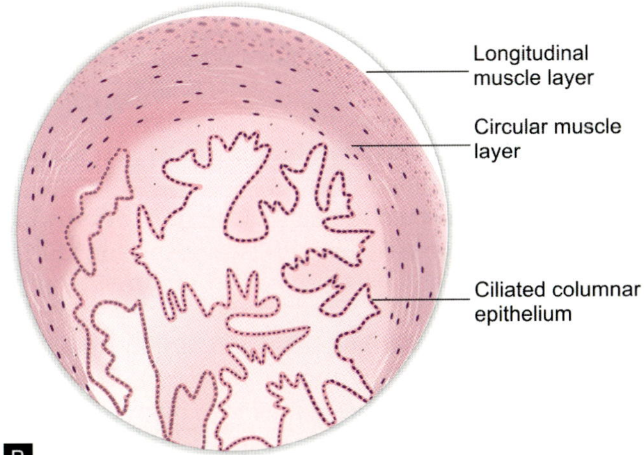

B

Figures 22.4A and B: Fallopian tube. **A.** Photograph; **B.** Diagrammatic representation.

- Name the different types of cells present in mucosa of fallopian tube.
- In which part of the fallopian tube does fertilization occur?

UTERUS (PROLIFERATIVE PHASE)

Slide No. 60

Identification Points

- Endometrium lined by simple columnar epithelium.
- Lamina propria containing uterine glands.
- Thick myometrium with numerous blood vessels.

Introduction

- Uterus (Figs 22.5A and B) is a pear shaped, thick muscular organ situated in the pelvic cavity
- It has fundus, middle body and lower cervix; out of which body forms the major part of uterus.

Structure

A detailed structure of proliferative phase of uterus can be explained as follows.

Endometrium: It is nothing but the mucosa of uterus:

- Endometrium is lined by simple columnar epithelium (it is ciliated before puberty)

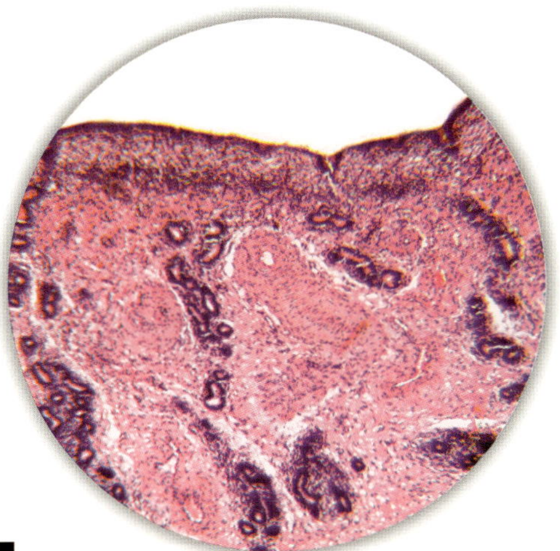

A

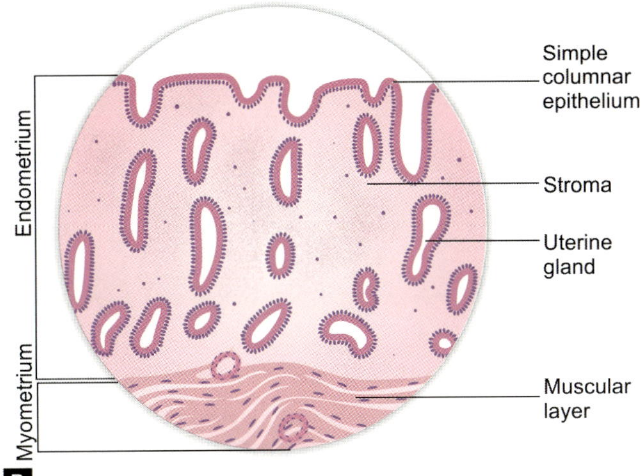

B

Figures 22.5A and B: Uterus (proliferative phase). **A.** Photograph; **B.** Diagrammatic representation.

- Just below the surface epithelium there exist stroma rich in connective tissue cells, blood vessels and lymphatics
- Numerous (simple tubular) uterine glands are seen in the stroma of uterus, which open perpendicular to the endometrial surface.

Here endometrium has two functional layers:

- **Stratum functionalis:** It is the superficial part forming two third of the endometrium:
  - It contains many uterine glands with spiral arteries in it
  - In a non-pregnant women this layer is shed out during menstruation and develops back on hormonal influences.
- **Stratum basalis:** It is the deeper part forming one third of endometrium:
  - It is also rich in uterine glands with many straight or basal arteries
  - This layer remains preserved during menstruation and gives rise to the stratum functionalis on hormonal influences.

Myometrium: It is found below the endometrium and consists of an indistinct inner longitudinal, middle circular and outer longitudinal muscle layers with an interstitial connective tissue and numerous blood vessels in it.

Perimetrium: It is the outermost layer consisting of mesothelium and connective tissue fibers, which blends with broad ligament of uterus.

Discussion

- Name the three layers of uterus.
- What is endometrium? What does it contain?
- What is stratum functionalis? What is its significance?
- What is stratum basalis? What is its significance?
- Describe the myometrium of uterus.
- What is perimetrium? What is it made up of?

UTERUS (SECRETORY PHASE)

Slide No. 61

Identification Points

- Thick endometrium lined by simple columnar epithelium
- Lamina propria containing tortuous glands and coiled arteries
- Myometrium with numerous blood vessels.

Histology of secretory phase of uterus (Fig. 22.6) is almost same as that of proliferative stage of uterus except few extra features in endometrium like:

- Stroma of endometrium increases in its thickness due to the deposition of glycogen and lipids.
- Uterine glands become larger in size and they become more tortuous. Its because of their extra growth in length, which exceeds the thickness of endometrium.
- More number of blood vessels appear in endometrial stroma which are also tortuous in nature because of its hypervascularization.

Note: During pregnancy, muscle fibers present in myometrium undergoe hypertrophy and hyperplasia with an increase in interstitial connective tissue.

Discussion

- List the differences between proliferative and secretory phase of uterus.
- Why the uterine glands and vessels become more tortuous in secretory phase of uterus?
- Is their any change in the myometrium of uterus during pregnancy?

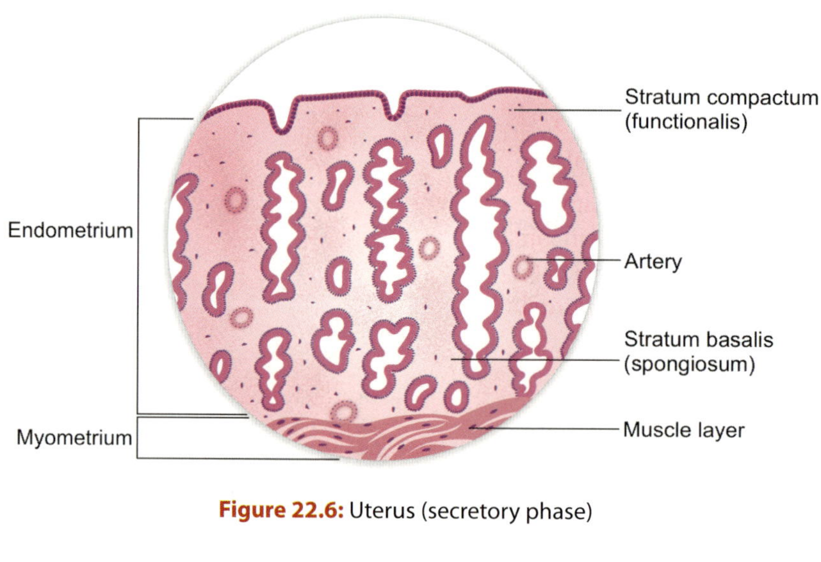

Figure 22.6: Uterus (secretory phase)

MAMMARY GLAND (LACTATING PHASE)

Slide No. 62

Identification Points

- Numerous prominent acinar lobules
- Acinar lobules lined by simple columnar epithelium
- Minimal connective tissue with duct system.

Introduction

- Mammary glands (Fig. 22.7) are the modified apocrine (sweat) glands situated in pectoral region
- They are rudimentary in males whereas in females they become prominent after puberty.

Structure

A detailed structure of lactating mammary gland can be explained as follows.

Parenchyma: Parenchyma of mammary gland is in the form of lobules:

- Parenchyma of lactating mammary gland is rich in lobules containing compound tubuloalveolar glands lined by simple columnar epithelium
- Here the surface epithelium of the glands are large and branched with an eosinophilic (milk) secretion in its lumen
- Here duct systems are not well-developed in lactating phase
- Numerous myoepitheliocytes are seen surrounding the glands on contraction of which, ejaculation of milk takes place.

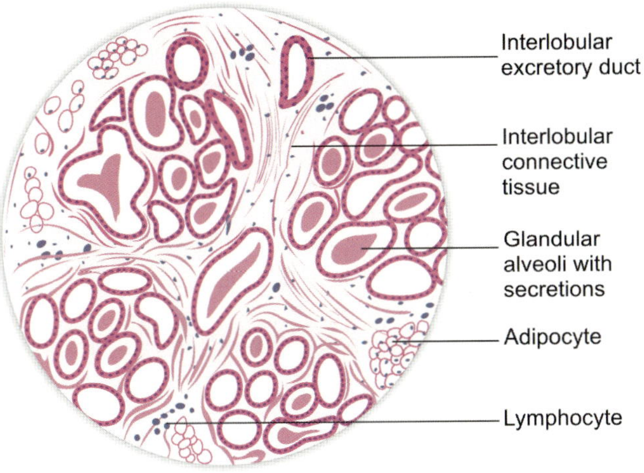

Figure 22.7: Mammary gland (lactating phase)

Stroma: It is made up of loose areolar connective tissue rich in adipocytes and fibers.

Amount of stroma in a lactating mammary gland is significantly decreased when compared to non-lactating mammary gland (Table 22.1).

Table 22.1: Differences between lactating and non-lactating mammary gland

Non-lactating mammary gland	Lactating mammary gland
Parenchyma is less	Parenchyma is more
Glands are lined by simple cuboidal or epithelium (low columnar epithelium)	Glands are lined by simple columnar
Glandular alveoli are small, its lumen does not contain anything	Glandular alveoli are large, its lumen contain eosinophilic (milk) secretin
Duct system is well-developed	Duct system is not well-developed
Stroma is more	Stroma is less
Stroma is rich in fibroblasts	Stroma contains few lymphocytes, plasma cells in it

Functions

- During lactation mammary gland secretes milk and nourishes the baby.

Discussion

- What is mammary gland? What type of gland is it?
- Name the surface epithelium covering the mammary gland?
- Enumerate the differences between non-lactating and lactating mammary gland.
- What is colostrum?

UMBILICAL CORD

Slide No. 63

Identification Points

- Two umbilical arteries
- One umbilical vein
- Wharton's jelly is present.

Umbilical cord (Fig. 22.8) is a long tubular structure connecting the fetus with placenta. A cut section of umbilical cord shows:

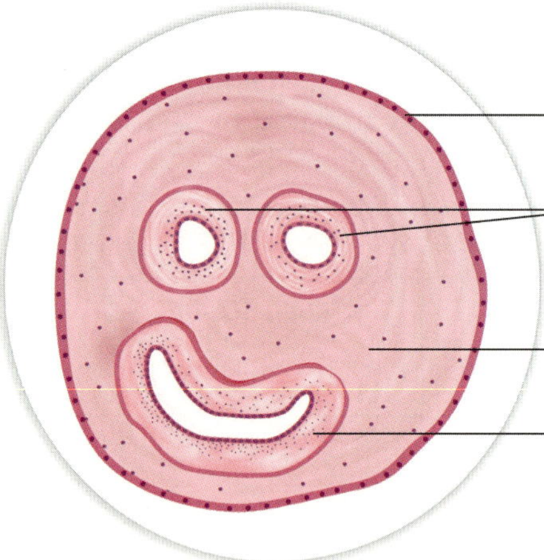

Figure 22.8: Umbilical cord

- Large amount of mucoid connective tissue or Wharton's jelly containing many star-shaped fibroblasts
- Umbilical vessels embedded in the substance of Wharton's jelly and the vessels are two umbilical arteries and an umbilical vein
- Amniotic epithelium surrounding the **Wharton's jelly** can also be seen.

Discussion

- What is an umbilical cord?
- What is Wharton's jelly?
- Which type of connective tissue is seen in umbilical cord?
- How many umbilical vessels are embedded in its connective tissue?
- Which is the outermost layer encircling the Wharton's jelly?

Chapter

23 Central Nervous System

INTRODUCTION

- Brain and spinal cord together form central nervous system (Fig. 23.1).
- Brain is further divided into forebrain, midbrain and hindbrain; whereas spinal cord is differentiated into cervical, thoracic, lumbar and sacral parts.

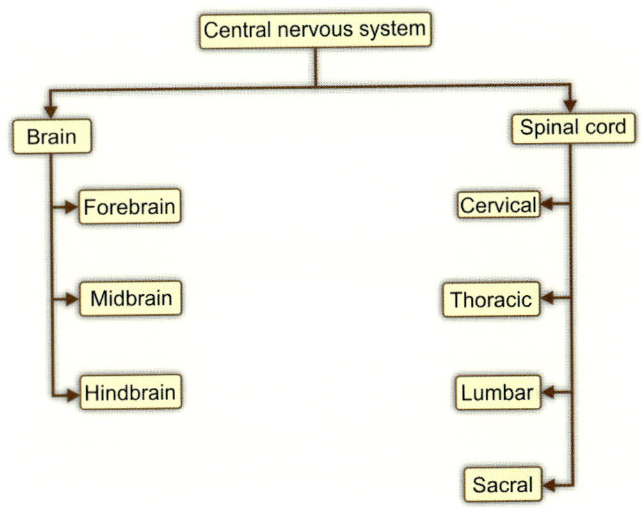

Figure 23.1: Classification of central nervous system

CEREBRUM

Slide No. 64

Identification Points

- Outer pia mater
- Six-layered cells are present
- Inner and outer bands of Baillarger are visible.

Structure

Histology of cerebral cortex shows following types of nerve cells arranged in six layers (Figs 23.2A and B). However, there is no clear-cut margin between the layers. The nerve cells of cerebral cortex are:

- Pyramidal cells
- Stellate (granule) cells
- Fusiform cells
- Horizontal cells of Cajal
- Cells of Martinotti.

The six different layers of cerebral cortex are:

- **Molecular layer (plexiform layer):** This is the most superficial and well-defined layer of cerebral cortex. It is made up of horizontal fibers of the axons of neuroglial cells and cells of Cajal.
- **External granular layer:** This layer contains large number of small pyramidal cells with few stellate cells and neuroglial cells.
- **External pyramidal layer:** It is made up aggregately of medium-sized pyramidal cells along with few stellate cells.
- **Internal granular layer:** This layer consists of densely packed stellate (granule) cells with few pyramidal cells and neuroglial cells. It contains a horizontal white fiber band called outer band of Baillarger.
- **Internal pyramidal layer:** It is also called ganglionic cell layer. It is made up of large pyramidal cells with few neuroglial cells. It also contains a horizontal white fiber band called inner band of Baillarger.
- **Multiform layer:** It is also called fusiform cell layer, as this layer predominates with fusiform cells.
  - Apart from this, it also contains intermixed cells of various size and shapes like stellate cells, spindle cells, cells of Martinotti and other neuroglial cells. Hence, it is also called pleomorphic layer.

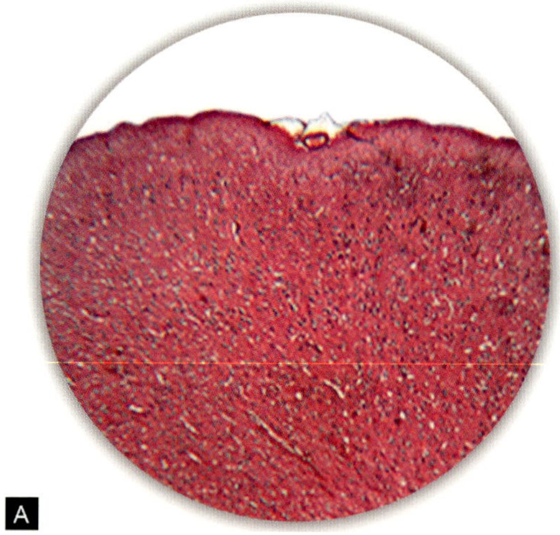

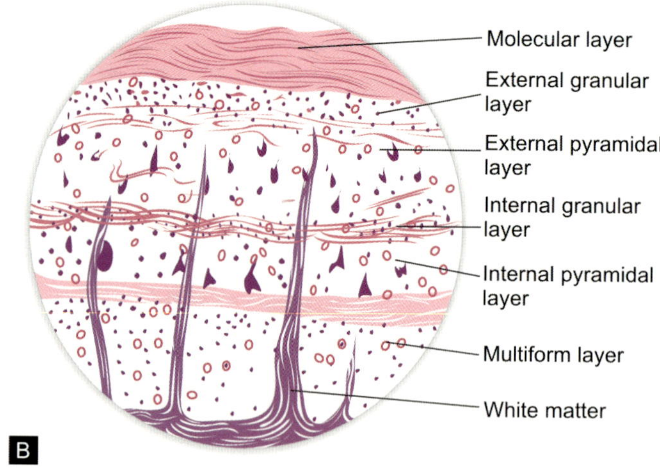

Figures 23.2A and B: Cerebrum. **A.** Photograph; **B.** Diagrammatic representation.

- Here few bundles of axons interrupt the cell layers and enter the white matter.

Discussions

- List the different types of cells present in gray matter of cerebral cortex.
- Enumerate the six layers of cerebral cortex.
- What is the another name for internal pyramidal layer?
- What are inner and outer bands of Baillarger?
- What is the other name for multiform layer? Why is it called so?

CEREBELLUM

Slide No. 65

Identification Points

- Outer molecular layer
- Middle Purkinje cell layer
- Inner granular layer.

Introduction

- Cerebellum is a cauliflower-shaped structure made up of many leaf-like processes called folia.

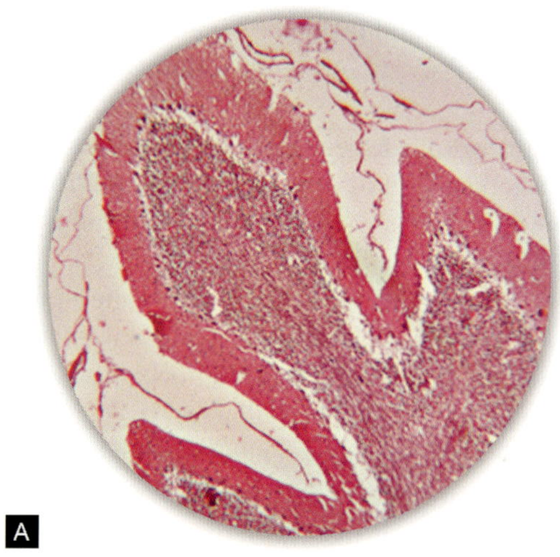

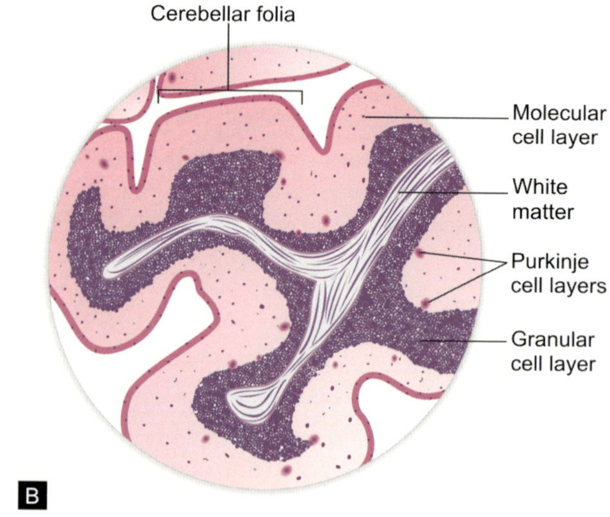

Figures 23.3A and B: Cerebellum. **A.** Photograph; **B.** Diagrammatic representation, showing three distinct layers.

- Each folia is differentiated into an outer cortex and inner medulla.
- Cortex of cerebellum is made up of gray matter where medulla has white matter in it.

Structure

Cortex: A detailed structure of cerebellar cortex shows three different layers and they are (Figs 23.3A and B):

- **Molecular cell layer:** It is the outermost layer of cerebellar cortex; appears light pink in color with routine hematoxylin and eosin (H and E) staining. It is made up of processes of stellate cells and basket cells, where stellate cells form the superficial layer and basket cells form deep layer.
- **Purkinje cell layer:** These are pear- or flask-shaped neurons found in between the molecular layer and granular cell layer. Since these cells are arranged in single layer, hence they are not so distinct, and axons of these cells penetrate the molecular layer.
- **Granular cell layer:** It is the innermost layer of cerebellar cortex, which is deeply stained by hematoxylin.
  - It is made up of densely packed small granule cells with darkly stained nuclei.
  - The dendrites and axons of these cells enter the molecular layer where they bifurcate into T-shaped manner.

Medulla: The medulla of cerebellar cortex is made up of white matter consisting of myelinated afferent and efferent nerve fibers of cerebellar cortex.

Discussions

- What are folia?
- Name the different layers of cerebellar cortex.
- What is molecular layer? What is it made up of?
- What does cerebellar medulla contain?

SPINAL CORD

Slide No. 66

Identification Points

- Outer white matter
- Inner H-shaped gray matter
- Central canal is present.

Structure

- Spinal cord (Fig. 23.4) is a part of central nervous system that lies in the upper two third of the canal in the vertebral column.
- Even though the basic structure of spinal cord is same all over, but it differs in its shape and structure with respect to the different levels in body.
- In general, transverse section of a spinal cord shows following structure.

White matter: It is the outer part of spinal cord rich in ascending and descending nerve fibers, i.e.:

- Nerve fibers of the white matter are preferably myelinated, which in formalin preserved; cut section appear white in color; hence it is called white matter.
- White matter of spinal cord is invaginated anteriorly by anterior median fissure and posteriorly by posterior median sulcus.
- Depending upon the site, white matter is divided into anterior white column, posterior white column and lateral white column.
- The nerve fibers of white matter are arranged into tracts. Based on its mode of action, they are classified into sensory and motor tracts.

Gray matter: It is the inner part of spinal cord rich in cell bodies of neurons, i.e.:

- On cut section, gray matter roughly resembles H-shape and is gray in color. Its gray color is due to non-myelination of cell bodies.
- Gray matter contains two anterior gray columns and two posterior gray columns.
- In a thoracic section of spinal cord, it also shows a lateral gray column on its either side.
- Both white matter and gray matter of spinal cord are differentiated in few aspects except its neuroglial cell, where both gray and white matter have same type of neuroglial cells.

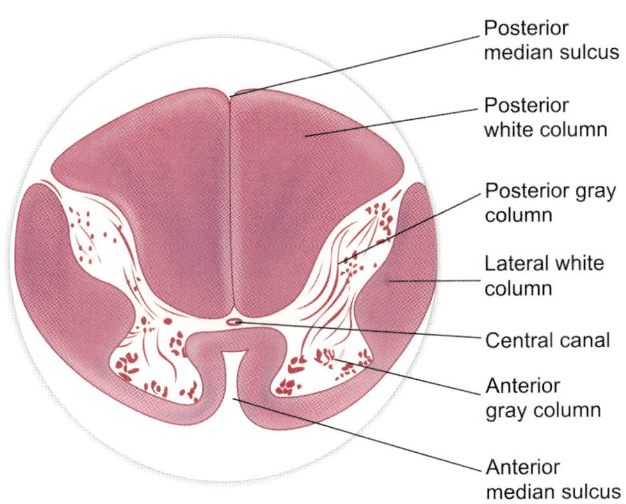

Figure 23.4: Spinal cord

Central canal: At the center of gray matter, there is small round canal-like structure called **central canal**. It is lined by ependyma and contains cerebrospinal fluid in it.

Discussions

- Name two distinct regions of spinal cord.
- What is white matter? What is it made up of?
- Name the different parts of white matter.
- What is gray matter? What is it made up of?
- Name the different parts of gray matter.
- In which segment of spinal cord you see lateral gray column?
- What is central canal? What does it contain?

Chapter

24 Organ of Special Sense (The Eye)

CORNEA (Figs 24.1A and B)

Slide No. 67

Identification Points

- Outer stratified squamous non-keratinized epithelium
- Intermediate stroma
- Inner endothelial lining.

Introduction

- Cornea is a transparent avascular structure forming anterior one sixth of the eyeball.
- Since it is avascular in nature, hence it gets its nutrition from its nearby structures and it is highly innervated by the nerve fibers.

Structure

A transverse section of cornea consists of five different layers and it is explained as follows:

- **Corneal epithelium:** It is the outermost layer of cornea lined by stratified squamous non-keratinized epithelium:
  - Here, the epithelium shows high capacity of regeneration with numerous microvilli on the superficial cell surface. They retain a thin film of **tear** (water) thus not allowing the cornea to dry out.
  - The epithelium of the cornea is highly sensitive because of numerous free nerve endings on it.
- **Anterior limiting (Bowman's) membrane:** It is a thick transparent homogeneous membrane seen just below the basement membrane of the corneal epithelium:

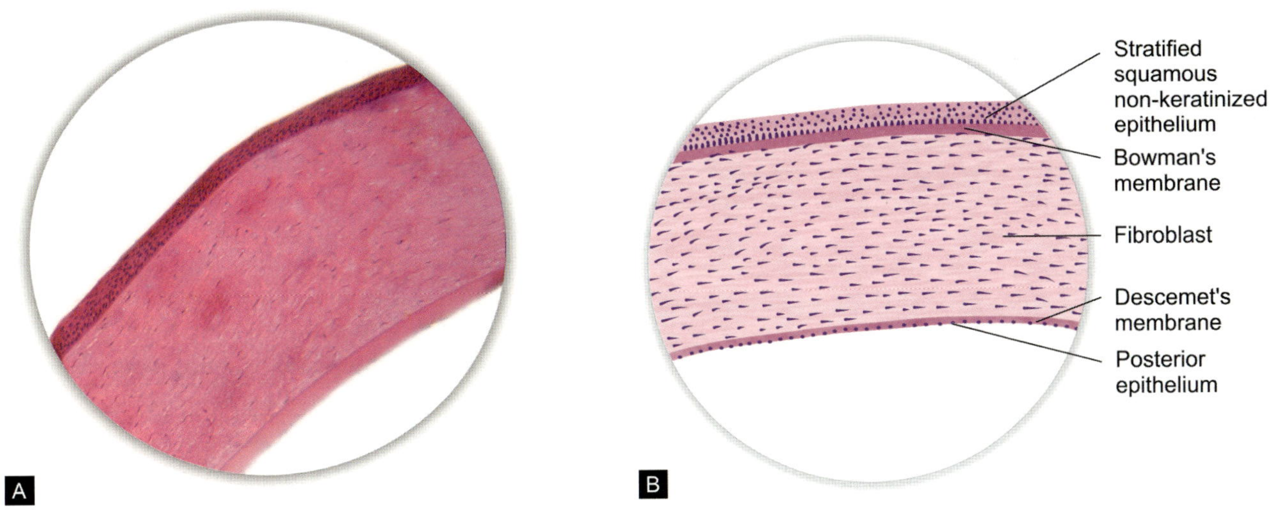

Figures 24.1A and B: Cornea. **A.** Photograph; **B.** Diagrammatic representation.

- It consists of compactly arranged collagen fibers, which gives a great support and strength to the cornel epithelium.

- **Stroma (substantia propria):** It forms the main bulk of the cornea constituting about 85%–90% of the total thickness:
  - It is made up of type II collagen fibers embedded in a ground substance rich in **sulfated glucosaminoglycans** such as chondroitin sulfate and keratin sulfate.
  - Here, the type II collagen fibers are arranged in the form of parallel lamellae with a uniform size and length with a same refractive index as that of ground substance, **hence the cornea appears to be very clear**.
  - Numerous star-shaped fibroblasts are also seen in the stroma of cornea which are also called **keratocytes** or **corneal corpuscles**.
- **Posterior limiting (Descemet's) membrane:** It is a thin transparent homogeneous membrane seen just below the stroma:
  - It consists of compactly arranged collagen fibers and is said to be the basement membrane of underlying epithelium.
- **Posterior epithelium:** It is the innermost layer of cornea made up of single layer of simple squamous epithelium resting on posterior limiting membrane:
  - It also forms the endothelium of the anterior chamber.

Functions

- Cornea plays a major role in refraction of light.
- Transparent nature of cornea allows the easy penetration of light into eye.
- It also protects the internal structure of the eyeball.

Clinical Histology
The tear layer present on cornea is rich in lysozymes, which act as an antibacterial agent, the absence of which leads to dryness of cornea, resulting in infections
Inflammation of the cornea is known as **keratitis** or **corneal ulcer** and most commonly it is caused by the bacterial agents, hence also called **bacterial corneal ulcer**
Surgical transplantation of the cornea is termed as corneal **keratoplasty**

Discussions

- What is cornea? Where is it located?
- List the different layers of cornea.
- Name the epithelium lining the corneal outer and inner surface.
- What is Bowman's membrane? What is its function?
- Name the type of collagen fibers seen in the stroma of cornea.
- What are keratocytes? What are its functions?
- Why is cornea transparent?
- Enumerate the functions of cornea.
- What is corneal ulcer?
- What is keratoplasty?

EYEBALL (RETINA) (Figs 24.2A and B)

Slide No. 68

Identification Points

- Outermost pigment cell layer
- Middle plexiform and nuclear layer
- Innermost internal limiting membrane.

Introduction

- An eyeball is made up of three layers; i.e. an outer **sclera**, middle **choroid** and inner **retina**.
- Sclera is rich in bundle of collagen fibers, fibroblasts with few melanocytes in its deeper layer, whereas choroid is further subdivided into suprachoroid lamina with melanocytes and vascular layer, choriocapillary layer, and transparent limiting membrane or glassy membrane **(Bruch's membrane)**.

Structure

A detailed structure of retina consists of 10 distinct layers, which can be explained as follows:

- **Pigment cell layer:** It is the outermost layer of retina made up of simple cuboidal epithelium with lots of pigments in it:
  - The base of the pigment cell layer rests on Bruch's membrane whereas its apex bears numerous processes, which extend into the rods and cones layer.
- **Layer of rods and cones:** It contains a layer of rod cells and cone cell, which are known as **photoreceptors**:
  - A rod cell is a modified neuron cell with long slender-shaped and rod-shaped process at its tip.
  - A cone cell is also a modified neuron cell with short, thick structure and a cone-shaped process at its tip.

  Here, the tips of rods and cones are surrounded by the processes of pigment cell layer.

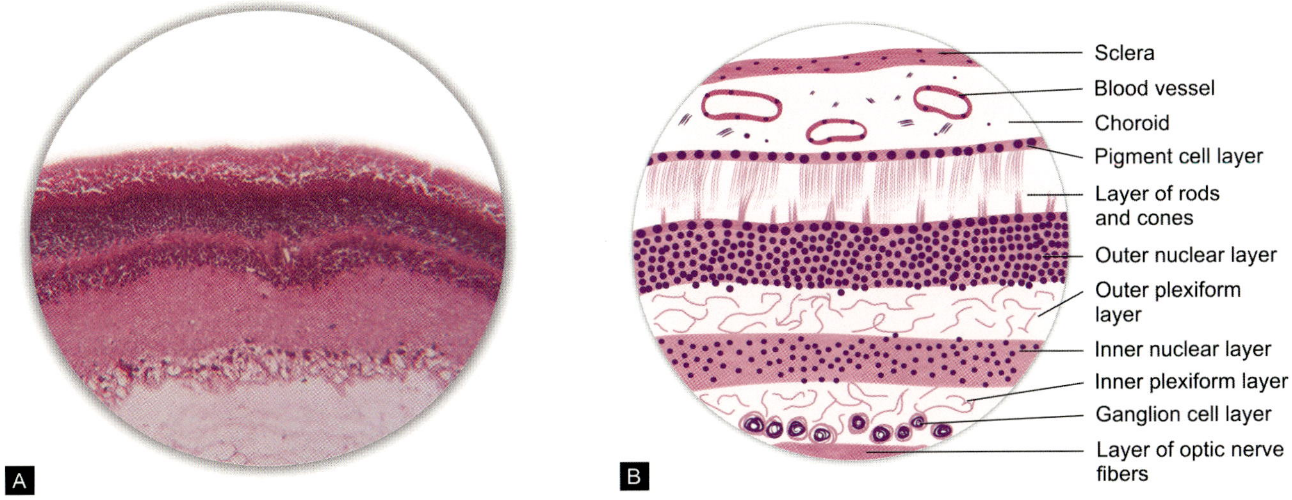

Figures 24.2A and B: Eyeball (retina). **A.** Photograph; **B.** Diagrammatic representation.

- **External limiting membrane:** It is a thin fenestrated membrane, which forms a series of junctional complexes between apices of **Muller's cells** and photoreceptors.
- **Outer nuclear layer:** This layer consists of cell bodies and nuclei of rod and cone cells. Here cone nuclei are close to the external limiting membrane than the rod nuclei.
- **Outer plexiform layer:** It is a synaptic zone consisting of axons of rods and cones with the dendrites of bipolar neurons, and process of horizontal cell therefore, it is also called **outer synaptic zone**.
- **Inner nuclear layer:** This layer contains the cell body and nuclei of bipolar neurons, horizontal **amacrine**, and **Muller's cells**.

  Here, bipolar cells are of two types:
  - Diffuse bipolar cells.
  - Monosynaptic bipolar cells.
- **Inner plexiform layer:** It is also another synaptic zone consisting of axons of bipolar neurons dendrites of ganglionic neurons and process of amacrine cells. Hence, it is also called an **inner synaptic zone**.
- **Ganglionic cell layer:** It is made up of bodies of ganglionic cells, with prominent euchromatic nuclei.

  Here ganglionic cells are of two types:
  - Midget ganglionic cells.
  - Polysynaptic ganglionic cells.
- **Nerve fibers layer:** This layer consists of axons of ganglionic cells, which pass through the lamina cribrosa of sclera to form optic nerve. Hence, some people refer this layer as **Stratum opticum**.
- **Internal limiting membrane:** It is the innermost layer of retina, which separates retina from vitreous:
  - It is formed by the union of terminal expansions of Muller's cells and their basement membrane.

Clinical Histology
Inflammation of the retina is called **retinitis**. The different types of retinitis are chorioretinitis, neuroretinitis and retinal vasculitis
Diabetic retinopathy is a microvascular complication of diabetes mellitus where in the vessels of retina are affected

Discussions

- Name the layers of retina.
- Which is the outermost and innermost layer of the retina?
- What is another name for outer plexiform layer? Why is it called so?
- What is stratum opticum?
- What are Muller's cells? In which layer do you see the terminal expansions of it?
- What is retinitis?

Index

Page numbers followed by *f* refer to figure and *t* refer to table.

D

E

F

G

H

I

J

K

L

M

N

O

P

R

S